Longevity and Geriatrics

Edited by Hülya Çakmur

Published in London, United Kingdom

Longevity and Geriatrics
http://dx.doi.org/10.5772/intechopen.1008034
Edited by Hülya Çakmur

Contributors
Alexandra Anatolyevna Melnichenko, Aryan Shukla, Eşref Selçuk, Francesca Morganti, Hilal Demirci, Howard R. Moskowitz, Jennifer Hanners Gutierrez, Jian Liu, Karen Samvelovich Bagdasaryan, Kepeng Ou, Larisa Viktorovna Girko, Li Zeng, Natalya Aleksandrovna Mokicheva, Neziha Erken, Seungwon Jeong, Sharon Wingert, Svetlana Girshevna Gorelik, Yanhong Fang, Yusuke Inoue

First published in London, United Kingdom, 2025 by IntechOpen
IntechOpen is the global imprint of INTECHOPEN LIMITED, registered in England and Wales, registration number: 11086078, 167-169 Great Portland Street, London, W1W 5PF, United Kingdom

For EU product safety concerns: IN TECH d.o.o., Prolaz Marije Krucifikse Kozulić 3, 51000 Rijeka, Croatia, info@intechopen.com or visit our website at intechopen.com.

British Library Cataloguing-in-Publication Data
A catalogue record for this book is available from the British Library

Longevity and Geriatrics
Edited by Hülya Çakmur
p. cm.
Print ISBN 978-1-83635-301-0
Online ISBN 978-1-83635-300-3
eBook (PDF) ISBN 978-1-83635-302-7

Meet the editor

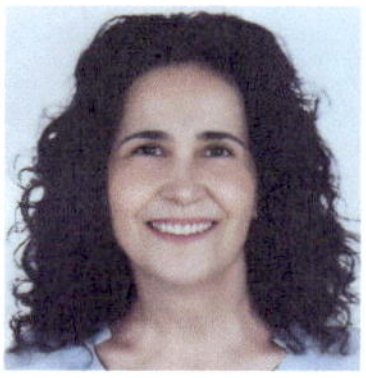

Hülya Çakmur graduated from the medical school at Atatürk University, Turkey. She completed her residency training in family medicine at Trakya University, Turkey. She obtained a Ph.D. in Public Health from Dokuz Eylül University, Turkey. She has 28 years of practice experience as a specialist in family medicine, including 15 years of experience in public health as a Ph.D.-prepared professional. She also studied sleep medicine at the University of Pittsburgh Medical Center in the USA and narrative medicine at St. Thomas University in Canada. She studied geriatrics voluntarily and published several studies in the field of geriatrics. She is an active member of the Turkish Medical Association and the European Academy of Teachers in General Practice/ Family Medicine. She has 14 years of experience as a professor at the University of Kafkas, Turkey, where she is the director of the Department of Family Medicine. She has published over fifty papers in reputable journals.

Contents

Preface

Understandably, conscious beings desire a long life. Throughout known human history, up to the present day, humankind has always sought long life, even immortality. At this stage, although more pronounced in developed countries, life expectancy at birth is increasing rapidly worldwide.

With the extension of life expectancy, the increase in aging and age-related health problems is inevitable. Aging is the primary risk factor for chronic diseases.

Age-related tissue and organ failure are among the most challenging issues facing modern medicine. This condition not only reduces an individual's quality of life and productivity but also accounts for a significant portion of healthcare expenditures. For this reason, healthcare policies are now focusing more on health span rather than lifespan. Health span, which refers to the practices aimed at living a healthy life, falls within the scope of longevity.

Longevity is a person-centered, holistic medical approach that aims to keep individuals healthy, productive, and disease-free throughout their lives by maintaining a youthful biological age. It seeks to protect and improve health by being proactive rather than reactive. To this end, it aims to prevent aging and chronic diseases by correcting many factors that are the root causes of aging and have been proven today (cellular, genetic, epigenetic, circadian rhythm, telomere loss, mitochondrial dysfunction, inflammation, dysbiosis, senescent cells, etc.).

The health problems experienced by geriatric individuals today, unfortunately, stem from the fact that innovations in the field of longevity have not been applied to these individuals.

When life spans are examined by country, it is evident that social determinants of health, such as socioeconomic status, education, a healthy environment, access to clean drinking water, and availability of healthy food, significantly impact life expectancy at birth. Therefore, regulating the social determinants of health is much more important than applying cellular and genetic interventions for longevity on an individual basis.

While presenting developments and applications in the field of longevity to the reader, this book also provides detailed information on the health problems faced by geriatric individuals and their solutions.

Hülya Çakmur
Kafkas University,
Turkey

Chapter 1

Community-Based Preventive Care in Japan: The Role of "Kayoi-no-ba" for Healthy Longevity among Older Adults

Seungwon Jeong and Yusuke Inoue

Abstract

Japan is the world's longest living country, yet the gap between life expectancy and healthy life expectancy remains approximately 10 years. This means that a substantial portion of older adults live with some degree of care dependency. While Japan's universal long-term care system provides comprehensive support for older adults, the increasing aging population and shrinking workforce pose serious challenges to the sustainability of this system. In response, many local governments have launched community-based preventive care programs aiming to extend healthy life expectancy and reduce the future burden of care. This chapter focuses on the local government-led preventive care initiative known as "Kayoi-no-ba," which provides older adults with regular opportunities for social participation and physical activity in community settings. Drawing on recent policy documents and empirical research, the chapter outlines the background, structure, and national promotion of "Kayoi-no-ba" programs. It also introduces key findings from studies evaluating their effectiveness in improving physical and mental health outcomes and preventing the progression of care needs among older adults. Through this analysis, the chapter sheds light on the practical potential and challenges of implementing community-based preventive strategies in an aging society like Japan.

Keywords: healthy aging, long-term care, long-term care prevention, "Kayoi-no-ba", older adults, Japan

1. Introduction

As of 2023, the number of older adults aged 65 and over in Japan was approximately 36.23 million, accounting for 29.1% of the total population. Among them, the population aged 65–74 comprised 13.0%, and those aged 75 and over comprised 16.1%. The aging rate varies across Japan's 47 prefectures, ranging approximately from 23 to 40% [1].

Japan is one of the countries with the highest life expectancy in the world. As of 2021, the average life expectancy was 81.7 years for men and 87.2 years for women, ranking among the highest globally. However, there is a significant gap between life expectancy and healthy life expectancy (i.e., years lived without limitations in daily activities or the need for long-term care). For both men and women, this gap is estimated to be around 10–12 years. As a result, many older adults spend their final years in a condition requiring some forms of assistance (**Figure 1**) [2].

This situation highlights the growing importance not only of living longer but also of maintaining physical and mental health, independence, and social engagement. Supporting older adults to live healthily and autonomously has become a key challenge for public policy and local communities in aging societies.

Since 2000, the population of older adults aged 75 and over in Japan has been steadily increasing (**Figure 2**). In particular, a sharp rise has been observed between

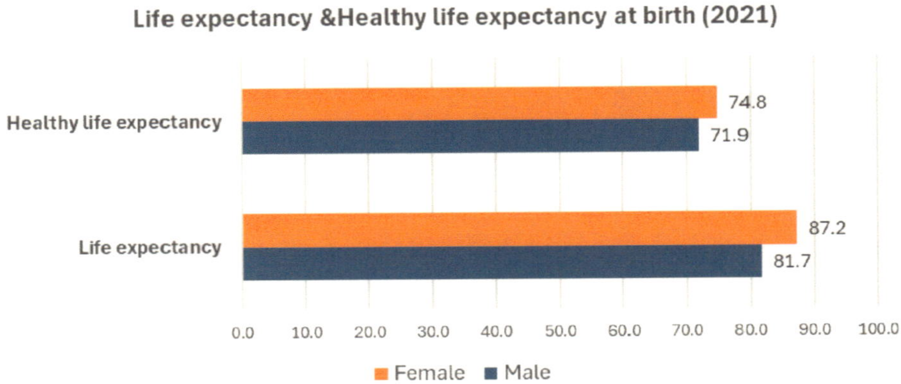

Figure 1.
Life expectancy and healthy life expectancy at birth. Data: OECD [2].

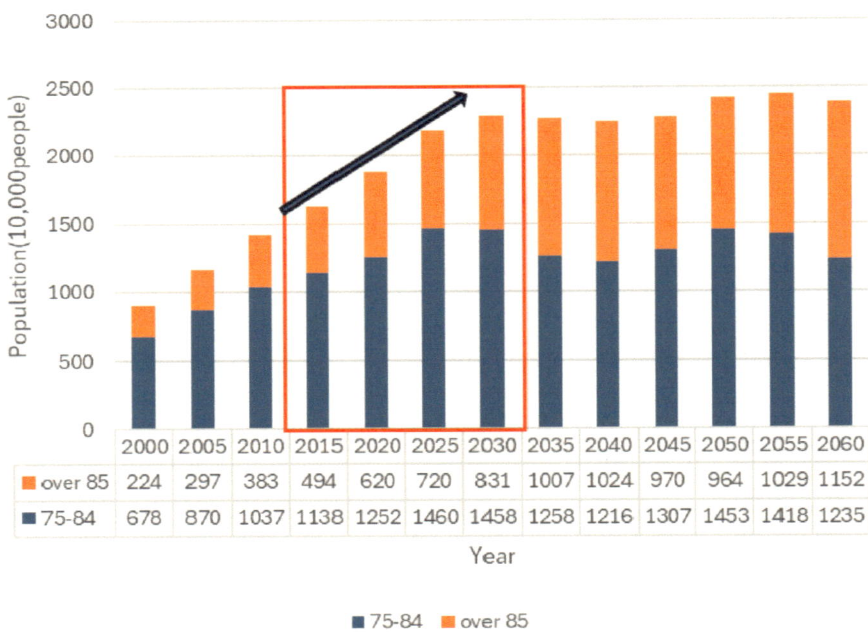

	2000	2005	2010	2015	2020	2025	2030	2035	2040	2045	2050	2055	2060
over 85	224	297	383	494	620	720	831	1007	1024	970	964	1029	1152
75-84	678	870	1037	1138	1252	1460	1458	1258	1216	1307	1453	1418	1235

Figure 2.
Population data for 2000–2020 are based on the Population Census; data for 2023 and 2024 are based on Population Estimates; and projections from 2025 onward are based on the Population Projections for Japan: 2023 Estimates [3].

2010 and 2030 [3]. This period coincides with the aging of the baby boomer generation—those born between 1947 and 1949—into the 75+ age group, raising concerns about a rapid surge in demand for medical and long-term care services.

The population aged 85 and over is expected to more than double, from approximately 3.8 million in 2010 to 8.3 million in 2030. This demographic shift underscores the critical importance of addressing the needs of the oldest-old in future policy planning. To meet these demands, continuous development of community-based support systems for older adults and the establishment of a sustainable healthcare and long-term care system are urgently required.

2. Long-term care insurance system and strategies for preventing dependency

Japan's social security system is a comprehensive framework composed of several pillars: the public pension system, health insurance system, long-term care insurance system, and employment insurance system. Collectively, these programs provide the foundational support for citizens' daily lives.

In response to the country's rapidly aging population, the Japanese government has identified the extension of healthy life expectancy among older adults as a key policy priority. Through initiatives such as Health Japan 21 (Second Term)—a national health promotion campaign—the government has aimed to strengthen community-based preventive health efforts. This includes disease prevention, the promotion of healthy lifestyles, and encouraging residents to take proactive roles in managing their own health.

Although Japan's healthcare and long-term care systems are internationally regarded as high-performing, demographic trends such as population aging, the shrinking working-age population, and rising costs of medical and long-term care services are placing increasing financial pressure on both national and local governments.

In this context, promoting "preventive care" for older adults—supporting them to remain healthy and independent for as long as possible—has become as important as the provision of medical and long-term care services themselves.

2.1 Long-term care insurance system

In response to the increasing number of older adults requiring care and the growing burden on families—such as due to the rise in elder-to-elder caregiving, where older individuals care for their elderly spouses or parents—Japan introduced the Long-Term Care Insurance (LTCI) system in 2000.

This system was established as a social mechanism to support care for older adults needs collectively across society.

The LTCI system rests on three core principles [4]:

First is "support for independence"—rather than simply providing care, the aim is to help older adults maintain as much independence as possible in their daily lives.

Second is "user-oriented service delivery," meaning that beneficiaries can choose from a range of services offered by various providers based on their own preferences and needs.

Third is the "social insurance model," wherein benefits and contributions are clearly linked under an insurance framework.

The system is funded equally by insurance premiums and public funds. Half of the financial resources come from insurance premiums paid by people aged 40 and older, and the other half from taxes contributed by the national, prefectural, and municipal governments.

Insured persons are divided into two categories:

- Category I (ages 65 and over): Premiums are generally deducted from pensions and collected by municipal governments.

- Category II (ages 40–64): Premiums are paid together with health insurance contributions and collected by health insurers.

When using LTCI services, users pay a copayment of 10% in principle, with higher-income individuals paying 20 or 30% depending on their income level [5].

2.2 Growth in the number of certified long-term care recipients

Since the implementation of the Long-Term Care Insurance system in 2000, the number of individuals certified as requiring long-term care has steadily increased in Japan. In FY2022, the total number of certified individuals reached approximately 6.94 million, which is about 3.2 times higher than in FY2000, when the system began with approximately 2.18 million (**Figure 3**) [6].

Among the certified, those categorized as "Care Level 1(the lowest level of formal care needs)" make up the largest share, followed by "Care Level 2", and then those in "Support Levels (mild level of need) 1 and 2." This trend indicates that a significant proportion of the certified population requires relatively mild-to-moderate assistance.

According to the data from FY2022, Support Levels 1 and 2 together account for about 20% of the total, while Care Levels 1 and 2 account for approximately 45%. These groups are therefore considered key targets for the long-term care prevention policies aimed at slowing the progression of care needs [6].

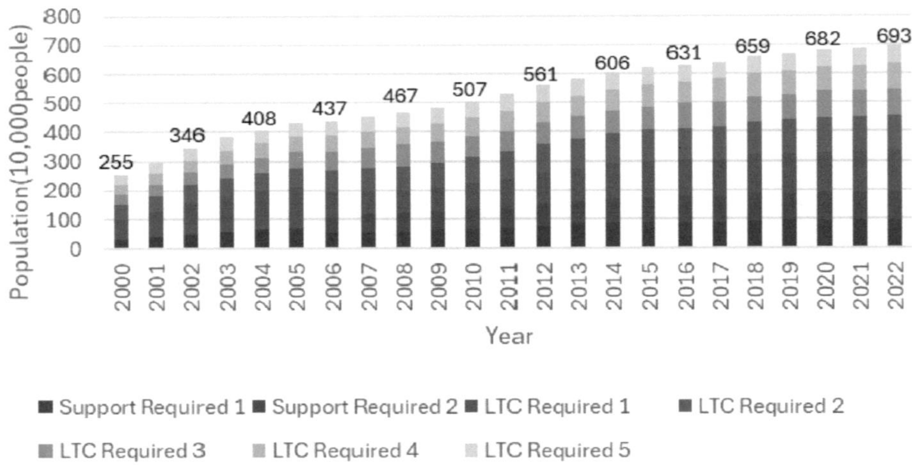

Figure 3.
Number of certified long-term care recipients. Source: Ministry of Health, Labour and Welfare (MHLW) [6].

2.3 Long-term care prevention

In rapidly aging Japan, long-term care prevention has become an urgent policy priority. The Ministry of Health, Labour and Welfare (MHLW) defines long-term care prevention not merely as improving physical functions such as mobility and nutrition, but as a broader concept:

"The goal is to enhance daily activity, encourage participation in family and social life, support individuals' sense of purpose and self-fulfillment, and thereby improve their quality of life" [7].

Effective long-term care prevention requires not only individual-level interventions such as physical rehabilitation, but also community-level approaches that improve the social and environmental contexts surrounding older adults. Based on this perspective, the Japanese government has promoted the development of community-based activities, particularly the establishment and expansion of "*Kayoi-no-ba*" (community gathering places), which are designed to be inclusive regardless of participants' age or physical condition [7].

Through these initiatives, the MHLW aims to build communities where social connections are strengthened and participation is encouraged, allowing these places and their users to grow and evolve together over time. In some municipalities, the positive outcomes of these efforts have begun to emerge, and expectations for local governments are increasing in terms of promoting long-term care prevention and community development.

To further support social participation, health maintenance, and prevention of care dependency among older adults, the MHLW promotes the development and utilization of "Kayoi-no-ba," where older adults can regularly engage in community activities in their daily lives.

In particular, providing spaces for relatively healthy older people to participate continuously in community-based activities is considered an effective means of delaying the onset of functional decline and reducing the risk of becoming dependent on long-term care.

3. Kayoi-no-ba (community gathering places)

3.1 The necessity of Kayoi-no-ba: From high-risk approach to population approach

In Japan, before the amendment of the Long-Term Care Insurance Act in 2014, preventive care programs were provided individually to older adults identified as being at high risk of needing long-term care [8]. This strategy was based on the high-risk approach. However, several issues became apparent, such as difficulties in identifying eligible individuals, low participation rates, and the inability of programs to meet the diverse needs of the target population [9].

In response to these limitations, Japan introduced a new policy direction in 2014 by establishing general preventive care services, including "Kayoi-no-ba." These services adopted a population approach, aiming to reach a broader segment of the older population through community-based comprehensive preventive strategies. This approach not only focuses on individual support but also emphasizes interventions that address the social and physical environments surrounding older adults.

3.2 What is Kayoi-no-ba and what activities are conducted?

"Kayoi-no-ba" refers to community-based gathering places where older adults can participate freely, regardless of their age or physical and mental conditions. These venues serve as hubs for a wide range of activities aimed at long-term care prevention and daily life support. Through local interactions in familiar settings, "Kayoi-no-ba" helps reduce social isolation and loneliness among older people, while also enhancing community safety, such as mutual aid during disasters and increased awareness of crime prevention.

The activities conducted at "Kayoi-no-ba" are diverse. They include physical exercises and fitness programs, hobby activities such as cooking classes and ground golf, agricultural work utilizing abandoned farmland, lifelong learning such as smartphone workshops, intergenerational exchanges in cooperation with children's cafeterias (community-based meal programs for children), and even employment-related programs. These activities are tailored to local characteristics and participant needs, providing participants with a sense of purpose and opportunities for self-fulfillment [10].

In recent years, efforts have been made to strengthen the functions of "Kayoi-no-ba" and ensure sustainable support. This includes the integration of health services and long-term care prevention, as well as the use of the Community Rehabilitation Activity Support Project which is a government initiative aimed at promoting rehabilitation and preventive care for older adults in community settings. Under these frameworks, professionals such as public health nurses, dietitians, and dental hygienists visit the venues to offer services like dementia prevention, nutritional counseling, and oral care.

3.3 Who operates Kayoi-no-ba, where, and how?

"Kayoi-no-ba" is a community-based initiative designed to promote daily interaction and health among older adults, based on their voluntary participation. Its management structures, locations, and activities vary widely [7].

The managing bodies include local residents themselves (volunteers or informal groups), neighborhood associations, non-profit organizations, municipal governments (especially long-term care prevention divisions), social welfare councils, healthcare institutions, care facilities, and private companies. Resident-led participation is regarded as essential, and professionals often support these activities in a supplementary role.

These gatherings are held in a wide range of locations. They include private homes, vacant houses, public community centers, school buildings, libraries, parks, unused spaces within hospitals or care facilities, and vacant commercial units in shopping streets. These venues are flexibly chosen by utilizing available local resources.

The activities themselves are also diverse, typically centered around physical exercises. Other examples include communal meals, tea gatherings, dementia prevention programs, farming, lifelong learning, volunteering, work-oriented programs, and intergenerational exchanges. These activities contribute not only to maintaining or improving physical function, but also to enhancing social connections and a sense of purpose in life [10].

All of these efforts align with the general requirements for "Kayoi-no-ba," such as holding activities at least once per week, ensuring resident-led management, allowing open participation, and maintaining records at the municipal level. A wide variety of stakeholders work in coordination to operate these initiatives as part of a comprehensive community effort.

3.4 Current status and activities of Kayoi-no-ba

The number of "Kayoi-no-ba" and their participation rates temporarily declined in 2020 due to the impact of COVID-19, but has since shown signs of recovery (**Figure 4**).

The main activities of "Kayoi-no-ba" vary in frequency. Approximately 40% are held once a week or more, around 20% are held two to three times per month, and about 30% are held only once a month. In terms of content, physical exercise programs (such as group gymnastics) are the most common, accounting for more than half of all activities. These are followed by hobby-related activities and social gatherings such as tea parties. In addition, some sites also conduct volunteer work and dementia prevention programs.

Participation rates in "Kayoi-no-ba" differ considerably across prefectures, ranging from 15.2% in the highest to 2.8% in the lowest, showing a regional variation of approximately 5.4 times.

As for participant demographics, women make up about 80% of all participants. Moreover, the proportion of participants aged 75 years and older has been increasing year by year, exceeding 70% of the total as of FY2022 [9].

3.5 Examples of Kayoi-no-ba implementation

"Kayoi-no-ba" programs aimed at preventing the need for long-term care are not simply spaces for social interaction. Rather, they have a clear objective: to help older adults maintain or improve their health and to delay the onset of functional decline that may lead to long-term care needs. Local governments across Japan have developed "Kayoi-no-ba" in diverse formats tailored to the characteristics and needs of each community (**Figure 5**).

For example, in one community, a resident-led "Kayoi-no-ba" is held weekly at the local community center. This program functions as a place for group exercise, cognitive training, and casual tea gatherings. The operation is mainly handled by community volunteers, while the municipal Community Comprehensive Support Center provides assistance and guidance.

In another case, a municipality has utilized vacant spaces in commercial facilities to offer preventive care classes, nutrition counseling, and health check-ups. These

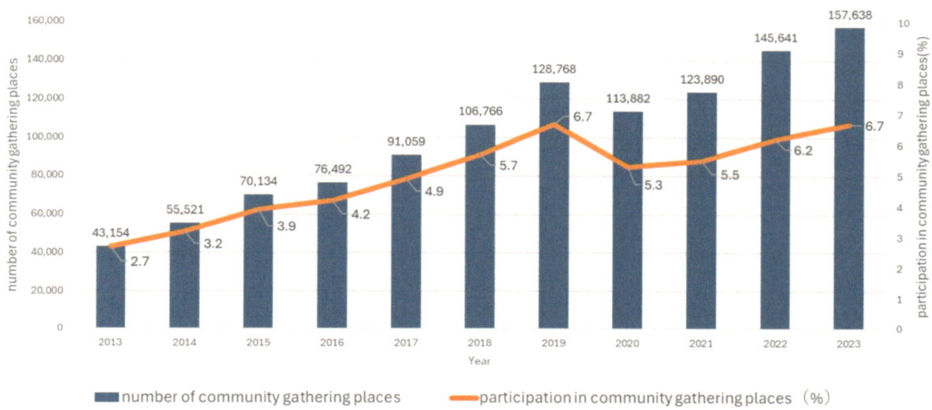

Figure 4.
Trends in the number of community gathering places and their participation rate. Source: Ministry of Health, Labour and Welfare, Manual for Addressing Issues in Community Gathering Places (Kayoi-no-ba), Ver.1, 2024.

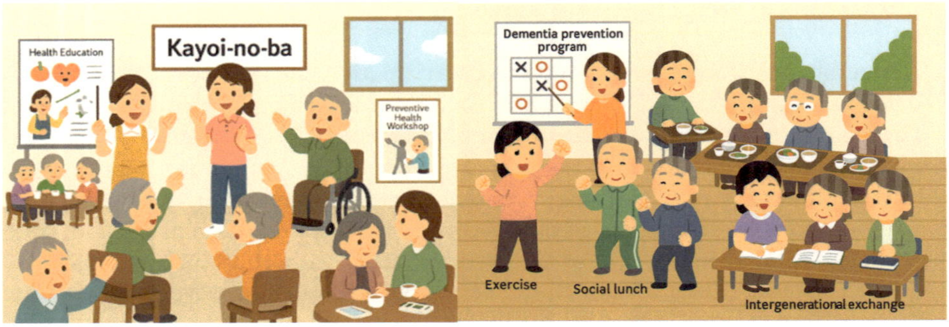

Figure 5.
Activities in Kayoi-no-ba.

efforts are often developed in partnership with private companies. Participants value the convenience and informal atmosphere, and such programs have become well-established as opportunities for regular social engagement.

Although the structure and content of "Kayoi-no-ba" differ from region to region, they consistently share three key features: (1) active participation by community residents, (2) utilization of local resources, and (3) ongoing support for sustainable operation. As such, "Kayoi-no-ba" are considered essential community strategies for extending healthy life expectancy and improving the quality of life (QOL) of older adults.

4. Evaluation of the effectiveness of Kayoi-no-ba

4.1 Why is it important to evaluate the effectiveness of preventive care?

The Ministry of Health, Labour and Welfare of Japan, in its report "Summary of Measures for Promoting General Preventive Care Services" [11], emphasizes the importance of measuring the effectiveness of preventive care as a part of the PDCA (Plan-Do-Check-Act) cycle for continuous program improvement.

In addition to its role in program management, effectiveness data can be used for multiple purposes.

- To visualize and confirm the outcomes of preventive care programs by local program managers.
- To ensure accountability when explaining results to local governments, assemblies, and community residents.
- To provide an evidence base for formulating future health and welfare plans.
- To support promotion efforts aimed at increasing program participation.
- To enhance participants' motivation for continued engagement.

Previous research suggests that if this cycle of planning, implementation, evaluation, and improvement functions well, it may lead to reduced growth in healthcare and long-term care expenditures in the medium to long term.

However, a prerequisite for this outcome is the systematic measurement and visualization of the program's effectiveness.

4.2 How are the effects evaluated?

The following datasets were collected from participating municipalities for analysis [12].

- Data from the Needs Survey in Daily Life Areas. This dataset includes information not only from older adults who participated in "Kayoi-no-ba" but also from non-participants. It provides comprehensive data on lifestyle habits, health-related indicators, social participation, and daily functioning. These variables are essential for assessing the differences between participants and non-participants and for conducting robust comparative analyses to evaluate the effectiveness of Kayoi-no-ba programs.
- Attendance records of participants in "Kayoi-no-ba" (at least two time periods)
- Long-term care certification records
- Mortality records
- Migration records (for residents who moved out)

Depending on the objective of the analysis, the following additional data may be integrated:

- Medical expenses data
- Long-term care expenditures
- Basic Checklist data (used for frailty and functional assessments in local governments)
- Other municipality-specific survey data

To rigorously examine the effects of preventive care programs, data are needed for both participants (intervention group) and non-participants (control group).

The outcome depends on several factors, including the magnitude of the program effect, the type of outcome variables used, and the length of follow-up. Thus, these figures should be regarded as general reference values [12, 13].

4.3 Methods

In the context of long-term care prevention programs, scientifically verifying the effects of interventions is critically important for ensuring policy validity and improving program quality. For "Kayoi-no-ba," a widely used evaluation method in existing research involves analyzing changes before and after program participation, targeting the participants themselves [8]. For example, changes in health-related indicators such as physical functioning, self-rated health, depressive symptoms, and nutritional status are typically assessed using descriptive approaches [13].

However, this before-and-after approach alone makes it difficult to determine whether the observed improvements are truly attributable to participation in "Kayoi-no-ba." This is because even older adults who do not participate may maintain or improve their health through other forms of community engagement or daily social activities. Therefore, to rigorously examine program effectiveness, it is necessary to compare outcomes between participants and non-participants [8, 12, 14].

Yet, a simple comparison between these two groups may introduce selection bias. Individuals who choose to participate in preventive care programs tend to be more health-conscious and socially active to begin with. As a result, comparisons with non-participants can create a false appearance of effectiveness that is actually due to these pre-existing differences.

The most scientifically valid approach to evaluate causality is the Randomized Controlled Trial (RCT), which randomly assigns individuals to intervention or control groups. However, in real-world community care settings, conducting RCTs is often difficult due to ethical and practical constraints.

To address this limitation, Propensity Score Matching (PSM) is commonly employed [15]. PSM is a statistical technique that matches individuals in the intervention and control groups based on background characteristics such as age, sex, medical history, and lifestyle. By comparing individuals with similar attributes, PSM helps reduce bias and allows for a more causal interpretation of program effects.

In observational studies of community programs like "Kayoi-no-ba," PSM has emerged as a practical and realistic method for evaluating effectiveness when randomized trials are not feasible.

4.4 Does "Kayoi-no-ba" effectively prevent care dependency?

A variety of indicators have been used to evaluate the effectiveness of community-based programs. Among them, physical functioning indicators such as walking speed, one-leg standing time, and physical fitness tests are the most frequently used. Other commonly used indicators include self-rated health, depressive tendencies (e.g., K6 scale), nutritional status, and levels of social participation. These are typically assessed using questionnaires, physical performance measurements, or validated screening tools.

Several types of programs have been reported to be associated with the positive outcomes in long-term care prevention, including the following (**Table 1**).

1. Health education programs focused on long-term care prevention and independence support, combined with professional counseling (e.g., by care managers), have shown improvements in mental health indicators such as the K6 score.

2. Fall prevention and dementia prevention programs have been associated with reductions in medical and long-term care costs, or the suppression of their growth.

3. Programs involving physical exercise, recreation, and handicrafts have been reported to contribute to the reduction of medical expenses.

4. Activities such as exercise, games, and intergenerational exchanges with preschool children have shown to reduce the risk of developing dementia and receiving long-term care certification.

5. Singing, playing musical instruments, and writing haiku poetry have contributed to improved self-rated health.

Reference	Sample size (n)	Observation period	Program contents	Main outcome indicators	Key findings
Yoshida et al. [16]	992 (Intervention group: 146, Control group: 846)	3 years	Fall prevention, dementia prevention	Medical and long-term care expenditures	In the intervention group, average monthly medical costs per person decreased, and long-term care costs slightly increased. In the control group, both medical and long-term care costs increased.
Ichida et al. [17]	1549 (Intervention group: 158, Control group: 1391)	8 months	Singing, musical instrument playing, haiku	Self-rated health	Participants in the intervention group were 2.52 times more likely to report better self-rated health compared to the control group.
Hikichi et al. [18]	2421 (Intervention group: 246, Control group: 2175)	5 years	Exercise, chatting, games, intergenerational exchange with preschoolers	Certification of need for long-term care	Intervention group showed a lower risk of receiving long-term care certification (7.7%) compared to the control group (14.0%).
Imahorii et al. [19]	409 (Intervention group: 157, Control group: 252)	1 year	Classes on prevention and independence support; consultations with professionals (care managers, public health nurses, dental hygienists)	Self-rated health, TMIG Index of Competence, K6 (psychological distress), outpatient visit status	Improvement in K6 scores in the intervention group.
Hikichi, et al. [20]	2007: 2593 (Intervention: 99, Control: 2494) 2010: 1769 (Intervention: 162, Control: 1607) 2013: 1352 (Intervention: 158, Control: 1194)	7 years	Exercise, chatting, games, interaction with preschool children	Incidence of dementia (Dementia Independence Level I)	Participation in "Kayoi-no-ba" (4+ times/year) reduced the risk of developing dementia to 0.7 times that of non-participants.
Ohtsuki [21]	1845 (Intervention: 721, Control: 1124)	2 years	Exercise, recreation, handicrafts, music, traditional cultural activities, interaction with children	Medical expenditure	Annual medical expenses per participant were ¥82,000 to ¥111,000 lower in the intervention group than in the control group.

Reference	Sample size (n)	Observation period	Program contents	Main outcome indicators	Key findings
Hosokawa et al. [22]	72 (Intervention: 16, Control: 56)	1 year	Sports activities, hobby activities, social tea gatherings	Functional ability (IADL and intellectual vitality)	Intervention group showed 1.2 times greater maintenance/ improvement in IADL and 1.3 times greater maintenance/ improvement in intellectual vitality compared to control group.
Tajika et al. [23]	3520 (Intervention: 472, Control: 3048)	3 years	Salon activities run by local governments or social welfare councils	Risk of requiring long-term care (Tsuji et al., 2018 scale) [24]	In the intervention group, the worsening of care-need risk score (≥5 points) was reduced by 46% among the oldest-old.
Abe et al. [25]	1239 (Intervention: 158, Control: 1081)	1 year	Genki Ouen Club (community-based activities: exercise, hobbies)	Risk of requiring long-term care (Tsuji et al., 2018 scale) [24]	Intervention group showed 28% lower risk deterioration after 1 year compared to control group.

Sources: Inoue et al. [12, 26].

Table 1.
Studies evaluating the preventive care effects of participation in "Kayoi-no-ba".

6. Participation in sports, hobbies, and tea gatherings has been shown to help maintain or improve functional capacity, including instrumental activities of daily living (IADL) and intellectual vitality.

7. Community-led activities have been associated with a lower risk of receiving certification for needing long-term care or support.

As a whole, many studies have reported improvements in physical function and subjective health as a result of these programs. However, findings regarding nutritional status are mixed; while some studies show improvement, others report no clear effect. These inconsistencies may reflect the diversity in program content, participant characteristics, and the lack of standardization in evaluation metrics and methodologies [12, 16–26].

Moreover, it is necessary to further examine how the frequency and intensity of program participation influence health outcomes. This remains a critical issue for future research to ensure the effectiveness and sustainability of long-term care prevention strategies.

5. Conclusions

This chapter has provided an overview of the role of "Kayoi-no-ba" in Japan's long-term care system and its potential for preventive care, especially in the context of an aging society.

Due to rapid population aging, extending healthy life expectancy has become a critical policy challenge in Japan. Since the 2014 revision of the Long-Term Care Insurance Act, a shift has been made from a high-risk approach to a population-based approach. As a result, "Kayoi-no-ba"—community-based gathering spaces—have been introduced and expanded nationwide.

"Kayoi-no-ba" serves as a hub for physical, psychological, and social well-being of older adults, offering programs such as exercise classes, hobby groups, and other social activities. These gatherings are primarily community-driven, utilizing local resources and tailored to the specific needs and characteristics of each area.

In evaluating the effects of "Kayoi-no-ba," it is not sufficient to rely solely on pre- and post-intervention comparisons among participants. More rigorous evaluations involving comparisons with non-participant groups are needed. Observational studies using techniques like propensity score matching have attempted to minimize bias and enable more causal interpretation. Research has also indicated that participation in "Kayoi-no-ba" may help suppress medical and long-term care expenditures and reduce the incidence of disability.

To improve the quality and sustainability of "Kayoi-no-ba," implementing the PDCA (Plan-Do-Check-Act) cycle is essential. Furthermore, the standardization and refinement of evaluation methods are important for evidence-based policymaking. The outcomes from such evaluations can also be used to:

- help local government officials monitor program effectiveness,
- fulfill accountability to the community,
- inform planning documents,
- promote program participation, and
- encourage continued engagement among participants.

6. Challenges of Kayoi-no-ba

Despite its benefits, "Kayoi-no-ba" still faces multiple challenges. These include a shortage of community leaders and supporters, difficulty in maintaining the continuity and quality of activities, and problems in attracting new and diverse participants.

At the administrative level, many municipalities lack adequate analysis of local needs and priorities, and there is limited understanding of effective strategies for operating "Kayoi-no-ba." Addressing these issues requires data-driven local assessments, strategic implementation planning, improved evaluation frameworks, stronger collaboration among stakeholders, and clear communication with residents.

In summary, for "Kayoi-no-ba" to continue serving as a central component of Japan's community-based integrated care system, it is vital to align data-based strategies at the policy level with flexible, community-led implementation on the ground.

Acknowledgements

This work was supported by the Japan Society for the Promotion of Science (JSPS) KAKENHI Grants-in-Aid for Scientific Research [Grant Numbers: 23K20654 and 22K02069].

Author details

Seungwon Jeong[1, 2*] and Yusuke Inoue[1]

1 Niimi University, Okayama, Japan

2 National Center for Geriatrics and Gerontology, Aichi, Japan

*Address all correspondence to: k-jeong@niimi-u.ac.jp

References

[1] Statistics Bureau, Ministry of Internal Affairs and Communications. Tokyo: Population Census; 2025. Available from: https://www.stat.go.jp/english/data/kokusei/index.html

[2] OECD. Life Expectancy at Birth (Indicator). OECD Health Statistics; 2023

[3] Statistics Bureau, Ministry of Internal Affairs and Communications. Elderly in Japan from the Viewpoint of Statistics. Tokyo: Statistics Bureau; 2024

[4] Ministry of Health, Labour and Welfare. Overview of the Long-Term Care Insurance System. 2021. Available from: https://www.mhlw.go.jp/content/001512842.pdf

[5] Ministry of Health, Labour and Welfare. Long-Term Care Insurance Business Report 2023. 2024. Available from: https://www.kaigokensaku.mhlw.go.jp/commentary/fee.html

[6] Ministry of Health. Labour and welfare. In: Annual Report on the Status of the Long-Term Care Insurance Project Report FY2022. Tokyo: MHLW; 2023. Available from: https://www.mhlw.go.jp/topics/kaigo/osirase/jigyo/22/index.html

[7] Ministry of Health, Labour and Welfare. Manual for Addressing Challenges in Kayoi-no-ba. Version 1. 2024. Available from: https://www.mhlw.go.jp/content/001244024.pdf

[8] Ministry of Health, Labour and Welfare. Guidelines for the Promotion of Integrated Community-Based Support Services for Preventive Care and Daily Life Support. 2nd ed. 2021. Available from: https://www.mhlw.go.jp/stf/seisakunitsuite/bunya/hukushi_kaigo/kaigo_koureisha/chiiki-houkatsu/index.html

[9] Ministry of Health, Labour and Welfare. Survey on the Progress of the Integrated Implementation of Health Projects and Preventive Long-Term Care Services for the Elderly. 2023. Available from: https://www.mhlw.go.jp/stf/seisakunitsuite/bunya/hukushi_kaigo/kaigo_koureisha/yobou/index.html

[10] Ministry of Health, Labour and Welfare. Survey Results on the Implementation of Comprehensive Community-Based Support Projects for Preventive Care and Daily Life Support (FY2022). Tokyo: MHLW; 2023. Available from: https://www.mhlw.go.jp/content/12300000/001417710.pdf

[11] Ministry of Health, Labour and Welfare. Summary of Measures for Promoting General Preventive Care Services. 2024. Available from: https://www.mhlw.go.jp/stf/seisakunitsuite/bunya/0000141576_00011.html

[12] Inoue Y, Jeong S, Ide K, Kondo K. Effects of "Kayoi-no-ba" for community-dwelling older adults: A systematic review. Chiiki Hoken. 2022;**53**(3):72-75 (in Japanese)

[13] Shinkai S et al. Public health approach to preventing frailty in the community: The Kihon checklist. Geriatrics & Gerontology International. 2016;**16**(Suppl 1):87-93. DOI: 10.1111/ggi.12701

[14] Takashima N et al. Impact of a population-based preventive home visit program on health-related quality of life among older adults. BMC Geriatrics. 2020;**20**(1):222. DOI: 10.1186/s12877-020-01613-2

[15] Rubin DB. Using propensity scores to help design observational studies:

Application to the tobacco litigation. Health Services & Outcomes Research Methodology. 2001;**2**(3-4):169-188. DOI: 10.1023/A:1020363010465

[16] Yoshida H, Fujiwara Y, Amano H, Kumagai O, Watanabe N, Lee SR, et al. Economic evaluation of preventive care programs: A comparative analysis of healthcare and long-term care costs between participants and non-participants. Japanese Journal of Public Health. 2007;**54**(3):156-167

[17] Ichida Y, Hirai H, Kondo K, Kawachi I, Takeda T, Endo H. Does social participation improve self-rated health in the older population? A quasi-experimental intervention study. Social Science & Medicine. 2013;**94**:83-90. DOI: 10.1016/j.socscimed.2013.06.006

[18] Hikichi H, Kondo N, Kondo K, Aida J, Takeda T, Kawachi I. Effect of a community intervention programme promoting social interactions on functional disability prevention for older adults: Propensity score matching and instrumental variable analyses, JAGES Taketoyo study. Journal of Epidemiology and Community Health. 2015;**69**(9):905-910. DOI: 10.1136/jech-2014-205345

[19] Imahori M, Izumita N, Shirase Y, Noguchi H. Empirical analysis of the effects of preventive care programs on physical and mental health: A case study of elderly salon in Abashiri City. Japanese Journal of Public Health. 2016;**63**(11):675-681

[20] Hikichi H, Kondo K, Takeda T, Kawachi I. Social interaction and cognitive decline: Results of a 7-year community intervention. Alzheimer's & Dementia: Translational Research & Clinical Interventions. 2017;**3**(1):23-32. DOI: 10.1016/j.trci.2017.01.002

[21] Ohtsuki T. Older community residents who participate in group activities have higher daily physical activity levels and lower medical costs. Asia-Pacific Journal of Public Health. 2018;**30**(7):629-634. DOI: 10.1177/1010539518805249

[22] Hosokawa R, Kondo K, Ito M, Miyaguni Y, Mizutani S, Goto F, et al. The effectiveness of Japan's community centers in facilitating social participation and maintaining the functional capacity of older people. Research on Aging. 2019;**41**(4):315-335. DOI: 10.1177/0164027519828066

[23] Tajika A, Ide K, Iizuka H, Tsuji T, Yokoyama M, Ojima T, et al. Does participation in "Kayoi-no-ba" suppress deterioration in long-term care needs? Longitudinal evidence from the JAGES 2013-2016 study. Japanese Journal of Public Health. 2022;**69**(2):136-145

[24] Tsuji T et al. Development of a risk assessment scale predicting incident functional disability among older people: Japan gerontological evaluation study. 2018. DOI: 10.1111/ggi.13503

[25] Abe N, Ide K, Tsuji T, Miyaguni Y, Sakuraba S, Kondo K. One-year effects of participation in community salons on long-term care needs: Longitudinal results from the JAGES Matsudo project. Sogo Rehabilitation. 2022;**50**(1):61-67

[26] Inoue Y, Jeong S, Ide K. Recommended sample size and observation period for evaluation. In: Kondo K, editor. The Development of "Kayoi-no-ba" in the Post-COVID Era. Tokyo: Japan Nursing Association Publishing Company; 2022. pp. 133-139 (in Japanese)

Chapter 2

Topical Therapies for Dry Age-Related Macular Degeneration on the Horizon

Li Zeng, Kepeng Ou, Yanhong Fang and Jian Liu

Abstract

With rising life expectancy, age-related diseases such as age-related macular degeneration (AMD) increasingly threaten the quality of life in older adults. This chapter contributes to the discourse on longevity and geriatrics by focusing on strategies to preserve vision, a key determinant of independence in aging populations. AMD, a progressive neurodegenerative retinal disease, is a leading cause of vision loss in the elderly. The dry form (dAMD), which accounts for 85–90% of cases, is marked by drusen accumulation beneath the retinal pigment epithelium (RPE), leading to RPE and photoreceptor degeneration. Its pathogenesis involves a multifactorial interplay of aging, genetic predisposition, oxidative stress, and immune dysregulation. Currently, there are no effective treatments for dAMD; anti-complement therapies for geographic atrophy (GA), the late stage of dAMD, have shown limited functional benefit in patients. Topical therapies offer promising advantages, including non-invasiveness, localized action, reduced systemic toxicity, and potential for cost-effective, patient-friendly interventions. However, developing effective eye drop formulations for dAMD remains a significant challenge, largely due to limited drug penetration to the posterior segment of the eye. Advances in understanding dAMD pathophysiology, coupled with novel delivery platforms, are essential to circumventing these barriers. A growing pipeline of small molecules and peptides targeting inflammation, autophagy, mitochondrial dysfunction, amyloid-beta toxicity, and choroidal circulation is currently under preclinical and clinical investigation. This chapter reviews the evolving therapeutic landscape for dAMD, emphasizing the potential of topical treatments to enhance patient care and support healthy aging.

Keywords: age-related macular degeneration, aging, neurodegeneration, retinal pigment epithelium, senescence, autophagy, inflammation, topical therapy, small molecules

1. Introduction

The ravages of aging without mitigation are embodied by the hapless mythical Greek prince Tithonus, who was loved by Eos, the goddess of the dawn. Driven by her desire to be with him forever, Eos asked Zeus to grant Tithonus eternal life, which was granted. To Tithonus's dismay, however, Eos forgot to ask for eternal youth. As time passed, he lived on and on but continued to age, eventually becoming so frail and incapacitated that he could no longer see, move, or speak.

Like Tithonus, people living longer today often face the burden of aging without preserving key functions such as vision. One of the clearest examples of this is vision loss due to age-related macular degeneration (AMD). AMD is a progressive and irreversible neurodegenerative disorder that has daunted many long before eternity, and it is the leading cause of vision loss in adults aged 50 and older. With increasing life expectancy, urbanization, and lifestyle changes, the global prevalence of AMD is projected to rise from the current 196 million to 288 million by 2040. This poses a growing burden on patients, healthcare systems, and society as a whole [1].

In 2020, the percentage contribution of AMD to all causes of blindness in individuals aged 50 and older ranged from 1.95% in Latin America and the Caribbean to 19.82% in high-income countries. Notably, while the estimated crude prevalence of AMD-related blindness globally decreased by 19.29% from 2000 to 2020, the prevalence of moderate and severe vision impairment (MSVI) increased by 10.08% [2]. This shift in the AMD severity profile may reflect advancements in diagnostic methods and anti-VEGF treatments for advanced neovascular AMD while simultaneously underscoring the lack of effective preventive and therapeutic options for early-stage AMD [3].

The landscape of topical therapies for retinal degenerations, including agents targeting AMD's pathogenic pathways and advances in ocular drug delivery, has been comprehensively reviewed elsewhere [4–7]. In this chapter, we focus specifically on dry AMD (dAMD), which accounts for 85–90% of all AMD cases, highlighting recent clinical trial outcomes and promising preclinical developments in topical treatment approaches.

2. Pathophysiology, challenges, and unmet needs in dAMD

AMD manifests in two main forms: dry (dAMD, also known as non-exudative or atrophic AMD) and wet AMD (exudative or neovascular AMD). dAMD is characterized by the accumulation of drusen, dysfunction of the retinal pigment epithelium (RPE), and loss of photoreceptors [1, 8]. A preclinical stage of AMD is defined by impaired dark adaptation in patients who present either no drusen or only small drusen and no pigmentary abnormalities. As dAMD progresses, it is further classified into early, intermediate, and advanced stages, with the latter known as geographic atrophy (GA) marked by outer retinal atrophic scars and photoreceptor cell loss. Sometimes, GA and neovascular AMD are jointly referred to as advanced AMD, as both represent late-stage disease associated with significant retinal damage, a high risk of central vision loss, MSVI, and legal blindness [9].

To understand how AMD undermines vision in aging individuals, it is essential to examine the cellular and molecular events that drive its progression. Genetic, metabolic, microvascular, inflammatory, and environmental factors all contribute to the complex mechanisms underlying AMD development. However, RPE cellular senescence and disrupted immune homeostasis are common threads that interconnect these critical biological processes [10, 11]. Aging, impaired autophagy, mitochondrial dysfunction, and recurrent or persistent oxidative stress can stimulate cellular senescence and promote the accumulation of senescent cells, which directly contribute to the formation of drusen and lipofuscin [12–15]. A subset of self-renewing RPE stem-like cells derived from human donors has been shown to acquire replicative senescence and a senescence-associated secretory phenotype (SASP). Higher levels of cellular senescence have been observed in AMD patients compared to healthy individuals [16]. The composition of drusen, including various lipids, proteins, and cellular debris, activates immune pathways of chronic inflammation and exacerbates oxidative stress. Meanwhile, a variety of molecules released via paracrine or autocrine SASP, such as proinflammatory cytokines, chemokines, growth factors, proteases, and extracellular vesicles, create a proinflammatory environment. This milieu fosters abnormal immune responses from microglia and promotes epithelial-mesenchymal transition (EMT) in RPE cells, ultimately leading to damage of the RPE and retinal tissue [17–19].

Current treatments for AMD are often plagued by high costs, injection-related risks, limited efficacy, and, in particular, a lack of strategies for early-stage intervention to prevent disease progression. Over the past two decades, a broad array of therapeutic regimens for wAMD has been developed, refined, and standardized. These include anti-VEGF agents to reduce abnormal vessel growth and leakage, as well as emerging therapies targeting alternative mechanisms, such as the anti-FGF2 agent umedaptanib pegol and gene therapies aimed at restoring the expression of endostatin and angiostatin [8]. In contrast, no definitive treatment currently exists for dAMD. Management strategies remain largely limited to general health promotion and nutritional supplementation, such as the Age-Related Eye Disease Study 2 (AREDS2) formula. While significant resources are being directed toward innovative strategies like gene and cell therapies, these treatments are unlikely to become mainstream in the near future due to their cost, invasiveness, and limited practicality for early intervention.

Topical drug delivery holds promise for dAMD because it enables targeted local treatment, reduced systemic toxicity, improved patient convenience, and compatibility with combination therapies. However, this route has been limited by low penetrability and absorption rate, largely owing to the eye's unique anatomical and physiological complexity. A deeper understanding of dAMD pathophysiology, coupled with advancements in drug delivery systems targeting the posterior segment, may pave the way for more effective treatments. Several small molecules and peptides are currently in preclinical or clinical trials, targeting interconnected aspects of dAMD progression, such as inflammation, autophagy dysfunction, and toxic amyloid-beta (Aβ) aggregates.

3. Therapeutic landscape and challenges in dAMD: Why do topical treatments matter?

Patients with dAMD often receive only nutritional supplementation from their physicians. The antioxidant vitamin formulations in the AREDS supplements and their modified extension, AREDS2, were developed to reduce the risk of AMD progression, particularly in patients with intermediate dAMD. The original AREDS formulation included vitamins C and E, copper, zinc, and beta-carotene. AREDS2 replaced beta-carotene with lutein and zeaxanthin, added omega-3 fatty acids (DHA and EPA), and reduced zinc content.

However, evidence regarding the efficacy of these supplements remains mixed, and the impact of targeted micronutrition may be confounded by overall dietary patterns. A recent study found that adherence to a Mediterranean-type diet (aMedi) was associated with a foveal-sparing effect and protection against proximity-based GA progression. Specifically, higher intake of vegetables and components of the aMedi diet was correlated with slower GA expansion and delayed central macular involvement in the AREDS or AREDS2 cohorts [20]. Conversely, a retrospective analysis of dAMD eyes without GA found that AREDS2 use was associated with an increased likelihood of incident GA, possibly reflecting confounding due to the strong correlation between intermediate AMD stage and AREDS2 usage [21]. Overall, neither AREDS nor AREDS2 has demonstrated confirmed efficacy in treating dAMD or significantly slowing GA progression. To further explore nutritional supplementation beyond AREDS2, a randomized phase 2 clinical trial (NCT05170048) is scheduled to begin in June 2025, evaluating AREDS2 plus the oral antioxidant EG-EPMP-01 (150 mg daily) in patients with non-foveal GA.

Beyond nutrition, pharmacological approaches, particularly anti-complement therapies, have shown limited success. Recent clinical trials have targeted the complement cascade, a key pathway in AMD pathogenesis. In 2023, pegcetacoplan (SYFOVRE) became the first Food and Drug Administration (FDA)-approved drug for GA treatment, followed by avacincaptad pegol (Izervay). These agents inhibit C3 or C5 proteins, preventing complement activation. While they reduced GA progression by approximately 20%, they did not improve visual acuity and may increase the risk of neovascular AMD [22]. Consequently, these therapies have not been approved by the European Medicines Agency (EMA) or the UK's Medicines and Healthcare Products Regulatory Agency (MHRA).

Other non-topical treatment strategies for dAMD include cell-based and gene therapies. In advanced dAMD, characterized by significant loss of RPE and photoreceptors, stem cell-derived retinal cell replacement has emerged as a potential approach. Various cell types, such as human embryonic stem cells (hESCs), induced pluripotent stem cells (iPSCs), and umbilical tissue-derived cells (hUTCs), have been studied for their ability to restore retinal structure and function. These differentiated retinal cells may be either delivered in suspension or seeded onto thin scaffolds to replace damaged tissue. Luxa Biotechnology recently reported preliminary results from a phase 1/2a clinical trial (NCT04627428) evaluating submacular transplantation of RPE stem cell-derived RPE cells (RPESC-RPE-4 W) in dAMD patients. Among six treated individuals, modest to substantial improvements in best-corrected visual acuity (BCVA) were observed, particularly in those with moderate to severe baseline vision impairment [23]. A meta-analysis of 12 cell therapy studies showed visual acuity improvements in both wAMD and dAMD; however, statistically significant reduction in logarithmic minimum angle of resolution (LogMAR) score was observed only in wAMD cases [24].

Gene therapy trials targeting multiple pathogenic mechanisms in dAMD are also underway. For example, a phase 3 trial (NCT06373731) is evaluating the subcutaneous injection of the mitochondria-targeted peptide Elamipretide, and the results are awaited. Additionally, a phase 2 trial (NCT05481827) and several phase 1/2 trials are investigating subretinal gene therapy approaches aimed at pathways involved in dAMD pathogenesis, including lipid metabolism, inflammation, oxidative stress, and complement activation [25]. Due to their complexity, invasiveness, and early development stage, these therapies are unlikely to be widely accessible to patients with early-stage dAMD in the near future.

Drugs for dAMD can be delivered via various routes: topical (eye drops), systemic (oral), intravitreal, subretinal, or suprachoroidal injections, as well as periocular methods such as subconjunctival, posterior juxtascleral, and transscleral delivery [26, 27]. Each method has distinct advantages and limitations. Among these, topical medications [28] are the most economical, convenient, non-invasive, and localized option, though they face challenges, primarily related to limited bioavailability in the posterior segment of the eye.

Ophthalmic topical treatments, primarily eye drops, are effective mainly for anterior segment diseases affecting the cornea, conjunctiva, iris, or ciliary body but are significantly limited in delivering therapeutic concentrations to the RPE and photoreceptors, the primary targets in dAMD [29]. Drug penetration is impeded by the long diffusion distance and multiple anatomical, physiological, and metabolic ocular barriers [30, 31]. To protect retinal integrity, the eye has evolved several anatomical barriers including the cornea, conjunctiva, and sclera, while the blood-aqueous barrier (BAB) and blood-retina barrier (BRB) further restrict molecular diffusion into retinal tissue [32].

Depending on a drug's lipophilicity and formulation, topically administered agents can reach the posterior tissues via three main routes: (1) transvitreal—through the cornea and aqueous chamber, penetrating the lens to reach the vitreous humor and retina; (2) conjunctival/scleral—diffusing across the conjunctiva, sclera, and choroid; and (3) cornea/scleral—diffusing laterally from the cornea to the conjunctiva [32, 33].

Although topical drugs can be absorbed at the ocular surface, only a small fraction (0.07–4.3% of the active pharmaceutical ingredient) reaches the aqueous humor, with even smaller amounts reaching the posterior segment where AMD pathology develops [30, 34]. Drug retention (residence time) in the eye is further compromised by protective mechanisms such as reflex blinking, nasolacrimal drainage, episcleral blood flow, and rapid intraocular convection from the ciliary body to Schlemm's canal [31, 35]. Despite these challenges, topical therapies for dAMD are under active investigation and development, with multiple approaches in early clinical or preclinical stages, as outlined below and in **Table 1**. Overcoming these barriers could establish

Primary target	Agent	Trial ID*/Model	Study Phase	Key Findings
Choriocapillaris atrophy	MC-1101	NCT01013376	Phase 1 (Completed)	No ocular or systemic adverse effects reported
		NCT01922128	Phase 1 (Completed)	No adverse effects
		NCT01601483	Phase 2/3 (Terminated)	No adverse effects; efficacy data not available
		NCT02127463	Phase 2/3 (Completed)	Outcomes pending
	Isopropyl Unoprostone	NCT01379560	Phase 2 (Completed)	Outcomes pending
Mitochondrial dysfunction	Elamipretide	NCT02314299	Phase 1/2 (Completed)	Data not available
Oxidative stress / Inflammation	OT-551	NCT00306488	Phase 2 (Completed)	Modest visual benefit; no significant structural change
		NCT00485394	Phase 2 (Completed)	No significant effect in GA progression

Primary target	Agent	Trial ID*/Model	Study Phase	Key Findings
Amyloid-b aggregation	MRZ-99030	NCT06659549	Phase 2 (Ongoing)	Study enrolling; results expected in 2027
5-HT1A Receptor	Tandospirone	NCT00890097	Phase 3 (Terminated)	No benefit over placebo
Autophagy activation	Trehalose	Mouse model	Preclinical	Protected RPE and photoreceptors from light-induced damage [12]
Apoptosis / Inflammation	6R-FBP	Mouse & rabbit models	Preclinical	Ameliorated $NaIO_3$-induced retinal degeneration [36]
Necroptosis	RIPK1 inhibitor	Rat, rabbit, & pig models	Preclinical	Preserved retinal function post-$NaIO_3$ insult [37]
TLR signaling	TDIP	Mouse model	Preclinical	Reduced photoreceptor loss and TLR-mediated inflammation [38]
Cell death	CK41016	Rat & rabbit models	Preclinical	Effective retinal distribution; interspecies variability noted [33]

**Detailed information on clinical trials is available at https://clinicaltrials.gov.*

Table 1.
Summary of Topical Treatments for Dry AMD in Clinical and Preclinical Studies.

topical therapies as a viable and scalable solution to the unmet needs of early-stage AMD, providing a non-invasive approach to preserving vision in aging populations.

4. Topical agents for treating dAMD in clinical studies

Emerging topical therapies for dAMD target diverse pathogenic mechanisms, including choroidal blood flow (ChBF) enhancement, neuroprotection, anti-inflammation, mitochondrial support, Aβ clearance, oxidative stress mitigation, autophagy enhancement, and inhibition of cell death. While clinical studies in topical senotherapeutics, such as senolytics or senomorphics, remain limited in dAMD [18], approaches that improve mitochondrial function and decrease oxidative stress may indirectly influence senescence-related pathways.

4.1 Improving choroidal circulation via MC-1101 and isopropyl unoprostone

Age-related decrease in choriocapillaris density and ChBF have been implicated in AMD, though whether these are causal or secondary to RPE and photoreceptor degeneration remains debated. Nevertheless, ChBF decline correlates with increasing AMD severity and drusen localization [39].

MC-1101, a topical hydralazine-based formulation, utilizes nitric oxide-mediated vasodilation to increase ocular perfusion. Originally FDA-approved for hypertension in 1997, it is now patented for ChBF enhancement in ocular conditions [6, 7].

Early-phase clinical trials (NCT01013376, NCT01922128) established safety and tolerability in both healthy individuals and patients with early dAMD, showing transient ChBF elevation without significant adverse effects [6, 40]. Phase 2/3 studies were performed in patients with mild to moderate dAMD (NCT01601483) and early to intermediate dAMD (NCT02127463); results show favorable tolerability with variable hemodynamic response.

Isopropyl unoprostone (IU), a synthetic prostaglandin analog, improves ChBF through multiple vasodilatory mechanisms: (a) activation of the Big Potassium (BK) channel leading to hyperpolarization of vascular smooth muscle cells; (b) dilation of choroidal vessels to improve microcirculation; and (c) inhibition of endothelin-1 (ET-1)-mediated vasoconstriction [41, 42]. Initially developed for intraocular pressure reduction, IU was evaluated in a 54-week pilot study for wAMD in Japan (UMIN000007881) and is currently under investigation for dAMD in a phase 2 trial (NCT01379560).

While retinal and choroidal vasoconstriction have been hypothesized to contribute to AMD pathogenesis, systemic vasodilators show inconsistent epidemiological associations with AMD. Notably, the Beaver Dam Eye Study, a 20-year longitudinal study involving 5924 adults, found that the use of vasodilator or antihypertensive medications, particularly oral nitroglycerin, was associated with a 72% increased risk of early AMD. No significant link between these medications and GA progression was observed [43].

4.2 Supporting mitochondrial function via Elamipretide

The retina's energy demands are among the highest in the body, rendering mitochondrial dysfunction a central feature of AMD pathogenesis [44]. Strategies such as photobiomodulation (PBM) and mitochondrial transplantation have shown preclinical efficacy in restoring mitochondrial activity, reducing inflammation, and clearing Aβ deposits [45–47].

Elamipretide (or MTP-131), a synthetic, cell-permeable tetrapeptide, targets cardiolipin in the inner mitochondrial membrane to stabilize electron transport and enhance bioenergetics. Despite its hydrophilicity, elamipretide can penetrate cell membranes and translocate into mitochondria due to its small size, aromatic chain, and catatonic nature. In dAMD murine models, systemic Elamipretide reduced oxidative stress and subretinal deposits [48].

A phase 2 trial (NCT03891875) in noncentral GA reported preserved ellipsoid zone (EZ) integrity after 48 weeks of subcutaneous dosing (40 mg daily) but did not meet primary endpoints for visual acuity or GA area change [49]. A phase 3 trial (NCT06373731) is currently evaluating efficacy over 96 weeks.

Topically, Elamipretide has shown visual function restoration in diabetic retinopathy mouse models. In mice with streptozotocin (STZ)-induced diabetic retinopathy, both topical ophthalmic-formulated solution (30 mg/ml) and subcutaneous injection of Elamipretide (1 mg/kg) significantly restored visual function, without systemic metabolic effects [50]. A phase 1/2 trial (NCT02314299) tested the safety and efficacy of low- and high-dose forms of topical Elamipretide, administered twice a day in subjects with diabetic macular edema (DME) and intermediate dAMD; results are pending.

4.3 Reducing oxidative stress and inflammation via OT-551

OT-551, a hydroxylamine prodrug, converts to TEMPOL, a stable nitroxide free radical, within the eye. This redox system provides catalytic antioxidant and anti-inflammatory activity. Intraperitoneal injection of OT-551 has been shown to protect RPE cells from acute light damage in a rat model [51].

Studies have shown that OT-551 eye drops rapidly penetrate the cornea and subsequently diffuse through the aqueous and vitreous humors or take the scleral route to reach the retina. The drug's tolerability was confirmed in a single-center, open-label phase 2 trial (NCT00306488) in which ten patients with GA received topical 0.45% OT-551 three times daily. Though a small improvement in BCVA was noted (+0.2 vs. -11.3 letters over 2 years), other functional and structural endpoints, including contrast sensitivity and GA progression, showed no significant difference [52]. A larger multicenter phase 2 study (NCT00485394) with 137 patients also failed to demonstrate efficacy in slowing GA progression, despite good tolerability [6, 53]. These findings highlight the need for further studies to conclusively determine the therapeutic efficacy of OT-551 in slowing GA progression.

4.4 Inhibiting integrin via Risuteganib

Risuteganib (ALG-1001) is a synthetic oligopeptide targeting integrin receptors implicated in angiogenesis, inflammation, and neurodegeneration [54–56]. In mouse models of dry eye disease (DED), topical Risuteganib reduced ocular surface inflammation by downregulating the expression of integrin αM and ß2 subunits, key mediators in C3-mediated inflammatory pathways. In clinical trials, topical Risuteganib was evaluated in DED patients using concentrations ranging from low (0.125%) to high (0.6%), administered as one drop twice daily for 12 weeks. All treatment groups demonstrated improvement, including increased TBUT (tear film breakup time), decreased SICCA dryness score, and improved VAS symptom index [55].

In a phase 2 trial (NCT03626636) involving patients with intermediate dAMD, intravitreal Risuteganib demonstrated encouraging results, with a significantly greater proportion of treated patients gaining ≥8 Early Treatment Diabetic Retinopathy Study (ETDRS) letters in best-corrected visual acuity (BCVA) compared to the sham group [57]. The FDA has granted Special Protocol Assessment (SPA) status for its phase 2b/3 development, which also includes evaluation of a topical formulation [58].

4.5 Inhibiting amyloid-beta aggregates via MRZ-99030

Multiple large-scale epidemiological studies have suggested a potential bilateral association between AMD and cognitive decline. Aβ accumulation, a hallmark of both AMD and Alzheimer's disease (AD), contributes to drusen formation and retinal neurodegeneration [59–64]. Experimental studies have shown that subretinal injection of Aβ peptide directly induces RPE senescence, secretion of SASP factors, and AMD-like retinal degeneration in mice [64].

MRZ-99030 is a dipeptide that reduces $A\beta_{1-42}$ oligomers by triggering a non-amyloidogenic pathway, forming benign, amorphous $A\beta_{1-42}$ assemblies [65]. It has also demonstrated the ability to reduce toxic Aβ species in the hippocampus, thereby reversing the synaptotoxic effects of Aβ oligomers in rat models [66]. MRZ-99030 operates via a unique self-propagating mechanism, whereby the administrated compound continues to gather and sequester misfolded Aβ monomers.

An MRZ-99030-derived ophthalmic solution named GAL-101 (2%) is currently in a phase 2 trial, eDREAM (NCT06659549), aiming to slow GA lesion expansion and photoreceptor degeneration over 12–24 months. The trial is estimated to enroll 110 participants and is expected to conclude in 2027.

4.6 Modulating serotonin receptors via Tandospirone

As a member of the G protein-coupled receptor family that binds the endogenous neurotransmitter serotonin (5-hydroxytryptamine, 5-HT), the 5-HT1A receptor is expressed in retinal tissues. 5-HT1A receptor has shown antioxidant and neuroprotective effects in oxidative stress models [67, 68]. In superoxide dismutase 2 (SOD2) knockout mice, which exhibit exaggerated oxidative stress and an AMD-like phenotype, daily subcutaneous 5-HT1A agonist, 8-OH-DPAT, exhibited antioxidant and neuroprotective effects, reducing lipofuscin accumulation and increasing photoreceptor survival.

Tandospirone, a selective 5-HT1A agonist primarily used as an antidepressant, exerts neuroprotective effects through 5-HT1A activation. Its topical formulation, AL-8309B (1% or 1.75% tandospirone), was developed for patients with GA (NCT00890097). Unfortunately, although no ocular adverse events were identified, GA lesion growth and mean visual acuity did not significantly differ between treatment and control groups [69], suggesting that broad serotonergic modulation may be insufficient to halt retinal neurodegeneration.

5. Topical agents for treating retinal degeneration in preclinical studies

Various synthetic or repurposed therapeutic agents have been evaluated as eye drops in preclinical models of dAMD (**Table 1**). Although these early efforts have not yet been brought under the scrutiny of clinical studies, their demonstrated efficacy in animal studies suggests promising avenues for future therapeutic development.

5.1 Inducing autophagy via trehalose

Autophagy is an essential catabolic process that mediates the degradation and recycling of damaged proteins, lipids, and organelles through lysosomal pathways. It plays a pivotal role in cellular homeostasis, especially in post-mitotic cells such as the RPE and photoreceptors. Disruption of autophagy contributes to dAMD pathogenesis through the accumulation of intracellular lipofuscin and extracellular drusen, mitochondrial dysfunction, and increased oxidative stress [70–73].

Trehalose, a naturally occurring nonreducing disaccharide of D-glucose, penetrates cells through fluid-phase endocytosis and can reach intracellular concentrations in the millimolar range despite its hydrophilicity [30, 74]. It is a potent mTOR-independent activator of autophagy, exerting neuroprotective effects in mouse models of lysosomal storage diseases and other neurodegenerative conditions [75]. Mechanistically, trehalose enhances transcription factor EB (TFEB), a master regulator of lysosomal biogenesis, thereby restoring lysosomal function independently of mTORC1 inhibition [76]. Since TFEB activation also helps inhibit oxidative stress-induced senescence and the SASP in auditory cells [77], it is plausible that trehalose may exert similar protective effects against premature senescence in RPE cells.

In apolipoprotein E (APOE)-deficient mice, a model of early AMD, oral trehalose treatment ameliorated retinal functional loss and reduced Bruch's membrane thickening [78]. Clinically, trehalose-containing eye drops (3% w/v), often combined with carboxymethylcellulose or sodium hyaluronate, are widely used in DED for their anti-inflammatory and osmoprotective properties [79–81]. Trehalose has demonstrated excellent safety even at concentrations up to 30% [82], highlighting its potential for high-dose or long-term ophthalmic use.

Our recent study demonstrated that topical application of 9% trehalose twice daily for 2 weeks protected against light-induced RPE and photoreceptor damage in mice, preserving outer nuclear layer thickness and junctional F-actin organization. Raman spectroscopy confirmed trehalose penetration into the posterior segment [12]. While lipophilic drugs typically cross the corneal epithelium barrier via the transcellular route, hydrophilic drugs, including trehalose, more plausibly reach posterior ocular tissues through lateral diffusion across conjunctival and sclera, followed by penetration through Bruch's membrane and RPE [31, 83]. These findings support the therapeutic potential of topical trehalose for addressing early autophagy dysfunction in dAMD.

5.2 Inhibiting apoptosis and inflammation via 6R-conjugated Fas-blocking peptide

The transmembrane glycoprotein Fas (CD95), a member of the tumor necrosis factor (TNF) receptor superfamily, is a key mediator of apoptosis and inflammation in various retinal diseases, including AMD. Fas activation triggers the extrinsic apoptotic pathway via caspase-8 and engages mitochondrial cell death via truncated BID (tBID), often accompanied by the release of inflammatory cytokines such as TNF-α and IFN-γ through NF-κB pathways. Oxidative stress and p53 activation further upregulate Fas in RPE cells, potentiating their sensitivity to apoptosis [36, 84].

A Fas-blocking peptide (FBP) conjugated with a cell-penetrating hexa-arginine (6R) sequence demonstrated robust retinal protection when administered topically in $NaIO_3$-induced dAMD models in mice and rabbits. The 6R-FBP reduced Fas expression, pro-inflammatory cytokine production, and macrophage infiltration while enhancing M2 macrophage polarization. Retinal integrity was preserved, as confirmed by optical coherence tomography (OCT) and fundus imaging [36]. These findings underscore the potential of 6R-FBP eye drops in modulating Fas-mediated apoptosis and inflammation in dAMD.

5.3 Inhibiting necroptosis via RIPK1-inhibitory compound

Necroptosis, a regulated form of necrotic cell death, is orchestrated by receptor-interacting protein kinase 1 (RIPK1), which interacts with RIPK3 and mixed-lineage kinase-like domain (MLKL) to execute inflammatory cell death. This pathway is activated in response to oxidative stress, inflammatory cytokines, and damage-associated molecular patterns (DAMPs), all of which are elevated in AMD [85, 86]. dsDNA, a drusen component, can trigger necroptosis via RIPK1-RIPK3-MLKL, and RIPK3 knockout mice are protected against AMD-like retinal degeneration and neuroinflammation [87].

In other animal species, including rats, rabbits, and pigs, $NaIO_3$ injection induced RIPK1-mediated necroptosis in RPE cells, recapitulating features of human dAMD. Treatment with a synthetic RIPK1-inhibitory compound (RIC) via eye drops potently suppressed catalytic activity of RIPK1, preventing RPE cell loss and maintaining retinal function, as demonstrated by fundoscopy and electroretinogram analyses. The study also confirmed excellent retinal penetration without evident retinal toxicity [37].

5.4 Attenuating inflammation via TIR-derived immunomodulatory peptides

Toll-like receptor (TLR) signaling, mediated by Toll/interleukin-1 receptor (TIR) domains, plays a critical role in the immune response by recognizing pathogen-associated molecular patterns (PAMPs) and DAMPs, which underpin the host defense against both external pathogens and endogenous cellular damage. Upon ligand binding, TLRs undergo oligomerization, leading to the recruitment of adaptor proteins such as MyD88 and TRIF through TIR-TIR domain interactions. These interactions trigger a signaling cascade involving pathways such as NF-κB, MAPK, and IRF, ultimately inducing the production of cytokines, interferons, and inflammatory mediators [13, 88, 89]. To modulate TLR signaling in chronic immune-related disorders, TIR-derived immunomodulatory peptides (TDIPs) have been developed to block TIR-TIR interactions.

In a $NaIO_3$-induced retinal degeneration model, topical administration of TDIP1 and TDIP5 preserved the integrity of photoreceptor segments and reduced ONL thinning. Photoreceptor cell death was significantly attenuated. The TDIPs demonstrated favorable pharmacokinetics, with half-lives of 6–48 hours, and effectively suppressed TLR-driven complement C3 upregulation [38]. These findings support the development of TDIPs as anti-inflammatory eye drops for retinal degeneration.

5.5 Inhibiting retinal cell death via CK41016 and SBL03

CK41016 is a small-molecule antioxidant with demonstrated protective effects in RPE cells under oxidative stress. While its mechanism of action is not fully elucidated, pharmacokinetic studies in rats and rabbits indicate selective distribution to the retina and choroid following topical administration, with retinal drug levels maintained for several hours post-dosing [33]. However, lower retinal delivery in rabbits than in rats suggests interspecies variability that warrants further investigation prior to human application.

SBL03, developed by SeaBeLife Biotech, is a topical ophthalmic gel targeting both necroptosis and ferroptosis. In animal models replicating key features of GA, repeated topical administration of SBL03 demonstrated significant protection of retinal structure and function. Assessments using electroretinography, OCT, and fundus autofluorescence indicated that SBL03 effectively reached retinal tissue and preserved visual function. A clinical trial for SBL03 is anticipated in 2026, marking it as one of the most advanced necrosis-inhibiting eye drop candidates in dAMD therapeutics [90].

6. Overcoming barriers in topical drug delivery

One of the most critical obstacles in the development of topical agents for dAMD is achieving effective drug delivery to the posterior segment of the eye. Conventional eye drops often fail to reach the intended target tissues, such as the RPE, lack sustained action, and do not provide sufficient therapeutic duration to halt the progression of AMD.

To address these limitations, a variety of advanced topical formulations and sustained-release delivery systems have been developed to enhance drug penetration into and retention within posterior ocular tissues. These include nanoparticle-based delivery platforms, emulsions, nanostructured lipid carriers, liposomes, niosomes, cyclodextrins, in-situ gels, and contact lens-based drug delivery technologies [27, 31, 32].

For instance, a hydrogel ring designed for topical delivery of ofloxacin significantly increased therapeutically relevant concentrations in the retina and choroid in rabbits [91]. A dexamethasone delivery system (Dex-DS) employing a drug-eluting contact lens achieved controlled and enhanced drug delivery to the retina, with the retinal drug concentrations 200 times higher than those achieved with hourly dexamethasone drops in rabbits [92].

Although aqueous vehicles are commonly used for eye drop formulations, novel lipid-based nanocarriers have gained attention due to their ability to enhance drug diffusion and bioavailability in preclinical studies [93]. Examples include annexin A5-associated liposomes [94], submicron-sized (100 nm) lipid emulsions [95, 96], nanoemulsified fingolimod [97], and polyethyleneglycolylated microemulsion [98].

In a phase 1/2 prospective interventional clinical trial, high-dose oral administration of lipophilic statin atorvastatin (80 mg daily) in 23 patients with dAMD characterized by soft, lipid-rich drusen led to regression of lipid deposits, with some patients experiencing mild improvements in visual acuity [99]. However, systemic drug delivery is often limited by the restrictive nature of the blood-retinal barrier (BRB), reducing therapeutic efficacy.

Given these limitations of systemic delivery, researchers engineered a novel eye drop formulation using atorvastatin-loaded solid lipid nanoparticles. This formulation significantly improved corneal penetration and drug stability, enabled successful delivery to the posterior eye, and demonstrated ocular safety across multiple animal models, including rats, rabbits, and pigs [100]. Ongoing innovations in the pharmaceutical design of eye drops are expected to yield more effective drug delivery systems capable of treating posterior segment diseases such as dAMD.

7. The importance of disease stage and drug specificity

Due to the dynamic nature of pathological mechanisms in AMD, it is essential to optimize therapeutic timing and target specificity for treatment success. Data from our research and other studies emphasize the critical importance of aligning drug administration with disease stage to maximize efficacy while minimizing side effects [12, 101].

For example, transcriptomic analyses of autophagy-lysosome pathway genes in the RPE/choroid across aging and AMD progression reveal distinct regulatory patterns [12]. While aging is associated with a predominant downregulation of autophagy-lysosome gene expression, AMD introduces additional complexity, exhibiting stage-dependent dysregulation. In early AMD, age-related autophagy decline is not adequately compensated under oxidative or metabolic stress, leading to impaired waste clearance and cellular dysfunction. As the disease progresses to the intermediate stage, marked by increasing RPE and photoreceptor cell death, the remaining viable cells may mount a compensatory upregulation of autophagy and lysosomal pathways in an effort to manage accumulated damage. However, this compensatory mechanism appears to deteriorate with further progression. Ultimately, in late-stage AMD (GA or wAMD), autophagy and lysosome pathways become bidirectionally dysregulated, accompanied by extensive and irreversible cell loss [12].

This progression underscores the therapeutic challenge: because photoreceptor degeneration is largely irreversible, interventions applied during the advanced stages of AMD are less likely to restore retinal architecture or function effectively. Hence, initiating treatments, particularly autophagy-enhancing therapies, during early disease stages may be crucial. Delayed intervention may not only be ineffective but also could potentially exacerbate degeneration or interfere with maladaptive cellular responses [101–103].

Moreover, drug responses can be highly dose- and context-dependent. Trehalose, for instance, promotes autophagy and may delay the onset of cellular senescence in RPE cells under oxidative stress. However, at higher concentrations, trehalose has been shown to induce a transient, reparative senescence-like phenotype in fibroblasts—potentially aiding tissue repair rather than merely preventing degeneration [104]. These findings highlight a possible dual function of trehalose, with its effects varying by both concentration and cell type. Whether trehalose exhibits similar dose-dependent effects in retinal tissues at therapeutic concentrations remains uncertain and requires further investigation.

8. Combination therapy

Given that AMD involves both localized retinal pathology and systemic factors, an integrated treatment strategy targeting both domains may be essential [14, 105, 106]. One notion is that AMD represents an ocular manifestation of systemic conditions, with progression exacerbated by factors such as obesity, metabolic syndrome, and aging. Although current evidence remains limited, emerging studies suggest that combining local and systemic therapeutic approaches could yield synergistic effects, offering a promising avenue for future treatment strategies.

For instance, a recent case report described significant improvements in a 73-year-old patient with dAMD following daily home-based PBM alongside consistent intake of AREDS-2 supplements [107]. PBM is a low-energy light therapy that meets the metabolic demands of RPE and photoreceptors by activating mitochondrial function and enhancing ATP production. Over an eight-month period, the patient experienced enhanced visual acuity from 20/30 to 20/20 in one eye, while the other eye stabilized at 20/25. Furthermore, a notable reduction in drusen volume and number was observed in both eyes, suggesting potential synergistic effects of combining light therapy with systemic antioxidants.

Both topical and oral administration routes are non-invasive and offer optimal patient adherence. For patients with comorbidities such as obesity or metabolic or cardiovascular conditions, combination therapies that address both ocular and systemic components may be beneficial. One such candidate is metformin, which exerts cytoprotective effects primarily by activating the AMP-activated protein kinase (AMPK) pathway, a key regulator in aging, as well as through AMPK-independent mechanisms that regulate autophagy, apoptosis, and cellular senescence [108].

Preclinical studies have shown that metformin directly inhibits angiogenesis in human retinal vascular endothelial cells and suppresses neovascularization and diabetes-induced retinal leukostasis in STZ mice [109]. Epidemiological evidence further supports its protective role: a meta-analysis of retrospective data indicated a reduced risk of AMD in individuals with diabetes who used oral metformin [110]. A more recent meta-analysis of 18 observational studies, including over 2.6 million individuals, reported a significant reduction in AMD risk among metformin users, with observed benefit in both diabetic and non-diabetic populations, despite substantial heterogeneity across studies ($I^2 = 90\%$) [111].

These findings support the hypothesis that combining oral metformin with topical therapies in early dAMD may enhance therapeutic outcomes through additive or synergistic mechanisms. To validate this strategy, rigorous randomized controlled trials are needed to assess efficacy, optimal dosing, and potential interactions in diverse patient populations.

9. Conclusions

Topical treatments that are both safe and effective remain the "holy grail" for managing early-stage AMD, a condition that leaves many patients living in fear of its progression to irreversible, vision-threatening forms. Among therapeutic candidates investigated in clinical and preclinical settings, repurposed compounds are particularly compelling due to their established safety profiles, affordability, and potential for expedited regulatory approval. As our understanding of disease mechanisms deepens, an increasing number of eye drop-based therapies, either as monotherapy or in conjunction with systemic treatments, are expected to emerge in the near future. Nonetheless, the complexity of dAMD pathophysiology and the difficulty of achieving sufficient drug bioavailability at the site of retinal degeneration continue to pose significant challenges. In dAMD, the retina endures a slow but relentless deterioration, reminiscent of the myth of Tithonus, a figure granted eternal life without eternal youth, condemned to a state of perpetual decline. Our quest for effective, localized, and non-invasive treatments seeks to rewrite that fate, aiming to slow or even halt retinal degeneration while preserving function. By intervening early and delivering therapies directly to the eye, we aspire not only to protect vision but also to support healthy aging.

Acknowledgements

This work was supported by Sight Research UK (SAC052, JL), Macular Society (2425-SC-01, JL), National Natural Science Foundation of China (82301244, KO), Natural Science Foundation of Chongqing, China CSTC (CSTB2024NSCQ-MSX0248, KO).

Conflict of interest

The authors declare no conflict of interest.

Author details

Li Zeng[1†], Kepeng Ou[2†], Yanhong Fang[3] and Jian Liu[4*]

1 Shanxi Academy of Medical Sciences, Taiyuan, China

2 College of Pharmacy, National and Local Joint Engineering Research Center of Targeted and Innovative Therapeutics, IATTI, Chongqing University of Arts and Sciences, Chongqing, Chineea

3 School of Medicine, Chongqing University Jiangjin Hospital, Chongqing University, Chongqing, China

4 Academic Unit of Ophthalmology, Translational Health Sciences, Bristol Medical School, University of Bristol, Bristol, United Kingdom

*Address all correspondence to: jian.liu@bristol.ac.uk

†These authors are contributed equally.

References

[1] Fleckenstein M, Schmitz-Valckenberg S, Chakravarthy U. Age-related macular degeneration: A review. JAMA. 2024;**331**(2):147-157

[2] Vision Loss Expert Group of the Global Burden of Disease, S., G.B.D. Blindness, and C. Vision impairment, global estimates on the number of people blind or visually impaired by age-related macular degeneration: A meta-analysis from 2000 to 2020. Eye (London, England). 2024;**38**(11):2070-2082

[3] Hernández-Zimbrón LF et al. Age-related macular degeneration: New paradigms for treatment and management of AMD. Oxidative Medicine and Cellular Longevity. 2018;**2018**:8374647

[4] Girgis S, Lee LR. Treatment of dry age-related macular degeneration: A review. Clinical & Experimental Ophthalmology. 2023;**51**(8):835-852

[5] Parmar UPS et al. Antioxidants in age-related macular degeneration: Lights and shadows. Antioxidants (Basel). 2025;**14**(2):152

[6] Fabre M et al. Recent advances in age-related macular degeneration therapies. Molecules. 2022;**27**(16):5089

[7] Sarkar A et al. Novel and investigational therapies for wet and dry age-related macular degeneration. Drug Discovery Today. 2022;**27**(8):2322-2332

[8] Spiewak D et al. Summary of the therapeutic options for patients with dry and Neovascular AMD. Journal of Clinical Medicine. 2024;**13**(14):4227

[9] Vyawahare H, Shinde P. Age-related macular degeneration: Epidemiology, pathophysiology, diagnosis, and treatment. Cureus. 2022;**14**(9):e29583

[10] Lee KS et al. Cellular senescence in the aging retina and developments of senotherapies for age-related macular degeneration. Journal of Neuroinflammation. 2021;**18**(1):32

[11] Ambati J, Atkinson JP, Gelfand BD. Immunology of age-related macular degeneration. Nature Reviews. Immunology. 2013;**13**(6):438-451

[12] Cox K et al. Age-associated decline in autophagy pathways in the retinal pigment epithelium and protective effects of topical Trehalose in light-induced outer retinal degeneration in mice. Aging Cell. 2025:e70081

[13] Liu J et al. Replenishing IRAK-M expression in retinal pigment epithelium attenuates outer retinal degeneration. Science Translational Medicine. 2024;**16**(750):eadi4125

[14] Handa JT et al. A systems biology approach towards understanding and treating non-neovascular age-related macular degeneration. Nature Communications. 2019;**10**(1):3347

[15] Liu J et al. Impairing autophagy in retinal pigment epithelium leads to inflammasome activation and enhanced macrophage-mediated angiogenesis. Scientific Reports. 2016;**6**:20639

[16] Lazzarini R et al. Effects of senescent secretory phenotype acquisition on human retinal pigment epithelial stem cells. Aging (Albany NY). 2018;**10**(11):3173-3184

[17] Li C et al. Age-related macular degeneration: A disease of cellular

senescence and dysregulated immune homeostasis. Clinical Interventions in Aging. 2024;**19**:939-951

[18] Chen Y et al. The role of retinal pigment epithelial senescence and the potential of senotherapeutics in age-related macular degeneration. Survey of Ophthalmology. 2025:S0039-6257(25)00053-0

[19] Liu J et al. Myeloid cells expressing VEGF and arginase-1 following uptake of damaged retinal pigment epithelium suggests potential mechanism that drives the onset of choroidal angiogenesis in mice. PLoS One. 2013;**8**(8):e72935

[20] Agron E et al. Relationships between diet and geographic atrophy progression in the age-related eye diseases studies 1 and 2. Nutrients. 2025;**17**(5):771

[21] Chan KS et al. Levodopa is associated with reduced development of new-onset geographic atrophy in patients with age-related macular degeneration. Eye and vision (London, England). 2024;**11**(1):44

[22] Csaky KG et al. Drug approval for the treatment of geographic atrophy: How we got here and where we need to go. American Journal of Ophthalmology. 2024;**263**:231-239

[23] Ilic D, Liovic M. Industry updates from the field of stem cell research and regenerative medicine in March 2025. Regenerative Medicine. 2025:1-9

[24] Khaboushan AS et al. Cell therapy for retinal degenerative disorders: A systematic review and three-level meta-analysis. Journal of Translational Medicine. 2024;**22**(1):227

[25] Trincao-Marques J et al. Gene and cell therapy for age-related macular degeneration: A review. Survey of Ophthalmology. 2024;**69**(5):665-676

[26] Jimenez-Gomez Y et al. Novel treatments for age-related macular degeneration: A review of clinical advances in sustained drug delivery systems. Pharmaceutics. 2022;**14**(7):1473

[27] Paliwal H et al. Novel approaches in the drug development and delivery Systems for age-Related Macular Degeneration. Life (Basel). 2023;**13**(2):568

[28] DeBoer CMT, Agrawal R, Rahimy E. Novel oral medications for retinal disease: An update on clinical development. Current Opinion in Ophthalmology. 2023;**34**(3):203-210

[29] Israilevich R, Mahmoudzadeh R, Salabati M. Narrative review-drug delivery in age-related macular degeneration. Annals of Eye Science. 2021;**6**:3

[30] Ramsay E et al. Selective drug delivery to the retinal cells: Biological barriers and avenues. Journal of Controlled Release. 2023;**361**:1-19

[31] Varela-Fernandez R et al. Drug delivery to the posterior segment of the eye: Biopharmaceutic and pharmacokinetic considerations. Pharmaceutics. 2020;**12**(3):269

[32] Wang Y, Wang C. Novel eye drop delivery systems: Advance on formulation design strategies targeting anterior and posterior segments of the eye. Pharmaceutics. 2022;**14**(6):1150

[33] Choi EJ et al. A novel eye drop candidate for age-related macular degeneration treatment: Studies on its pharmacokinetics and distribution in rats and rabbits. Molecules. 2020;**25**(3):663

[34] Samoila L et al. Topical treatment for retinal degenerative pathologies: A systematic review. International Journal of Molecular Sciences. 2023;**24**(9):8045

[35] Yasukawa T, Ogura Y. Medical devices for the treatment of eye diseases. Handbook of Experimental Pharmacology. 2010;**197**:469-489

[36] Yi Y et al. Eye drop with Fas-blocking peptide attenuates age-related macular degeneration. Cells. 2024;**13**(6):548

[37] Jang KH et al. Protective effect of RIPK1-inhibitory compound in in vivo models for retinal degenerative disease. Experimental Eye Research. 2019;**180**:8-17

[38] Lim Y et al. Massively parallel screening of toll/Interleukin-1 receptor (TIR)-derived peptides reveals multiple toll-like receptors (TLRs)-targeting immunomodulatory peptides. Advanced Science (Weinh). 2025;**12**(1):e2406018

[39] Fragiotta S et al. Choroidal vasculature changes in age-related macular degeneration: From a molecular to a clinical perspective. International Journal of Molecular Sciences. 2022;**23**(19):12010

[40] Ralston P Jr et al. A pilot, open-label study of the safety of MC-1101 in both normal volunteers and patients with early nonexudative age-related macular degeneration. Investigative Ophthalmology & Visual Science. 2010;**51**(13):913

[41] Shiragami C et al. Effect of topical isopropyl unoprostone on macular atrophy progression in eyes with exudative age-related macular degeneration. Medicine (Baltimore). 2017;**96**(12):e6422

[42] Tsuruma K et al. Unoprostone reduces oxidative stress- and light-induced retinal cell death, and phagocytotic dysfunction, by activating BK channels. Molecular Vision. 2011;**17**:3556-3565

[43] Klein R, Myers CE, Klein BE. Vasodilators, blood pressure-lowering medications, and age-related macular degeneration: The beaver dam eye study. Ophthalmology. 2014;**121**(8):1604-1611

[44] Ji MH et al. The present and future of mitochondrial-based therapeutics for eye disease. Translational Vision Science & Technology. 2021;**10**(8):4

[45] Rassi TNO et al. Photobiomodulation efficacy in age-related macular degeneration: A systematic review and meta-analysis of randomized clinical trials. International Journal of Retina and Vitreous. 2024;**10**(1):54

[46] Noh SE et al. Inhibition of cellular senescence hallmarks by mitochondrial transplantation in senescence-induced ARPE-19 cells. Neurobiology of Aging. 2023;**121**:157-165

[47] Noh SE et al. Mitochondrial transplantation attenuates oligomeric amyloid-beta-induced mitochondrial dysfunction and tight junction protein destruction in retinal pigment epithelium. Free Radical Biology & Medicine. 2024;**212**:10-21

[48] Cousins SW et al. Mitochondrial dysfunction in experimental mouse models of SubRPE deposit formation and reversal by the Mito-reparative drug MTP-131. Investigative Ophthalmology & Visual Science. 2016;**57**(12):2126

[49] Ehlers JP et al. ReCLAIM-2: A randomized phase II clinical trial evaluating Elamipretide in age-related macular degeneration, geographic atrophy growth, visual function, and ellipsoid zone preservation. Ophthalmology Science. 2025;**5**(1):100628

[50] Alam NM et al. A mitochondrial therapeutic reverses visual decline

in mouse models of diabetes. Disease Models & Mechanisms. 2015;**8**(7):701-710

[51] Tanito M, Li F, Anderson RE. Protection of retinal pigment epithelium by OT-551 and its metabolite TEMPOL-H against light-induced damage in rats. Experimental Eye Research. 2010;**91**(1):111-114

[52] Wong WT et al. Treatment of geographic atrophy by the topical administration of OT-551: Results of a phase II clinical trial. Investigative Ophthalmology & Visual Science. 2010;**51**(12):6131-6139

[53] Sternberg P et al. Topical OT-551 for treating geographic atrophy: Phase II results. Investigative Ophthalmology & Visual Science. 2010;**51**(13):6416

[54] Kuppermann BD. A dual-mechanism drug for vitreoretinal diseases. Retina Today. 2015;**10**:85-87

[55] Lindstrom R et al. Safety and efficacy of ALG-1007 topical ophthalmic solution: A synthetic peptide that regulates inflammation, in patients with dry eye disease: An exploratory phase I, open-label, single-center clinical study. American Journal of Ophthalmic Clinical Trials. 2020;**3**:10

[56] Wu T, Liu C, Kannan RM. Systemic dendrimer-peptide therapies for wet age-related macular degeneration. Pharmaceutics. 2023;**15**(10):2428

[57] Boyer DS et al. Safety and efficacy of intravitreal risuteganib for non-exudative AMD: A multicenter, phase 2a, randomized, clinical trial. Ophthalmic Surgery, Lasers and Imaging Retina. 2021;**52**(6):327-335

[58] Allegro Ophthalmics L. Allegro Ophthalmics Receives FDA Agreement under Special Protocol Assessment (SPA) for Phase 2b/3 Clinical Trial of Risuteganib for the Treatment of Intermediate Dry AMD. 2023. [Internet]. Available from: https://www.seabelife.com/en/dry-amd-seabelife-achieves-highly-promising-preclinical-efficacy-results-for-sbl03-without-injections-into-eye/ [Accessed: May 12, 2025]

[59] Marchesi N et al. Ocular neurodegenerative diseases: Interconnection between retina and cortical areas. Cells. 2021;**10**(9):2394

[60] Gollisch T, Meister M. Eye smarter than scientists believed: Neural computations in circuits of the retina. Neuron. 2010;**65**(2):150-164

[61] Jiang Y et al. Outer retinal thinning is associated with brain atrophy in early age-related macular degeneration. American Journal of Ophthalmology. 2025;**269**:457-465

[62] Jabbehdari S et al. Age-related macular degeneration and neurodegenerative disorders: Shared pathways in complex interactions. Survey of Ophthalmology. 2024;**69**(3):303-310

[63] Anderson DH et al. Characterization of beta amyloid assemblies in drusen: The deposits associated with aging and age-related macular degeneration. Experimental Eye Research. 2004;**78**(2):243-256

[64] Liu C et al. Subretinal injection of amyloid-beta peptide accelerates RPE cell senescence and retinal degeneration. International Journal of Molecular Medicine. 2015;**35**(1):169-176

[65] Nashine S. Potential therapeutic candidates for age-related macular degeneration (AMD). Cells. 2021;**10**(9):2483

[66] Rammes G et al. MRZ-99030 - A novel modulator of Abeta aggregation: II - Reversal of Abeta oligomer-induced deficits in long-term potentiation (LTP) and cognitive performance in rats and mice. Neuropharmacology. 2015;**92**:170-182

[67] Thampi P et al. The 5HT1a receptor agonist 8-oh DPAT induces protection from lipofuscin accumulation and oxidative stress in the retinal pigment epithelium. PLoS One. 2012;**7**(4):e34468

[68] Biswal MR et al. Systemic treatment with a 5HT1a agonist induces anti-oxidant protection and preserves the retina from mitochondrial oxidative stress. Experimental Eye Research. 2015;**140**:94-105

[69] Jaffe GJ et al. Randomized trial to evaluate Tandospirone in geographic atrophy secondary to age-related macular degeneration: The GATE study. American Journal of Ophthalmology. 2015;**160**(6):1226-1234

[70] Chang KC et al. The interplay of autophagy and oxidative stress in the pathogenesis and therapy of retinal degenerative diseases. Cell & Bioscience. 2022;**12**(1):1

[71] Hyttinen JMT et al. Autophagy in drusen biogenesis secondary to age-related macular degeneration. Acta Ophthalmologica. 2024;**102**(7):759-772

[72] Zhang Z et al. Autophagy in dry AMD: A promising therapeutic strategy for retinal pigment epithelial cell damage. Experimental Eye Research. 2024;**242**:109889

[73] Blasiak J et al. Cellular senescence in age-related macular degeneration: Can autophagy and DNA damage response play a role? Oxidative Medicine and Cellular Longevity. 2017;**2017**:5293258

[74] Zhang M et al. Combining endocytic and freezing-induced trehalose uptake for cryopreservation of mammalian cells. Biotechnology Progress. 2017;**33**(1):229-235

[75] Lotfi P et al. Trehalose reduces retinal degeneration, neuroinflammation and storage burden caused by a lysosomal hydrolase deficiency. Autophagy. 2018;**14**(8):1419-1434

[76] Ghosh S et al. The AKT2/SIRT5/TFEB pathway as a potential therapeutic target in non-neovascular AMD. Nature Communications. 2024;**15**(1):6150

[77] Suzuki Y et al. Premature senescence is regulated by crosstalk among TFEB, the autophagy lysosomal pathway and ROS derived from damaged mitochondria in NaAsO(2)-exposed auditory cells. Cell Death Discovery. 2024;**10**(1):382

[78] Vessey KA et al. Treatments targeting autophagy ameliorate the age-related macular degeneration phenotype in mice lacking APOE (apolipoprotein E). Autophagy. 2022;**18**(10):2368-2384

[79] Ballesteros-Sanchez A et al. Trehalose and dry eye disease: A comprehensive systematic review of randomized controlled trials. Journal of Clinical Medicine. 2023;**12**(23):7301

[80] Bedei A et al. Real-world treatment outcomes of an artificial tear containing arabinogalactan, hyaluronic acid and Trehalose among subjects with dry eye. Clinical Ophthalmology. 2025;**19**:83-91

[81] Morya AK et al. Randomized controlled trial of trehalose: An efficient autophagic bioprotectant in the management of dry eye disease. Taiwan Journal of Ophthalmology. 2021;**11**(2):161-167

[82] Laihia J, Kaarniranta K. Trehalose for ocular surface health. Biomolecules. 2020;**10**:5

[83] Hughes PM et al. Topical and systemic drug delivery to the posterior segments. Advanced Drug Delivery Reviews. 2005;**57**(14):2010-2032

[84] Zacks DN et al. Cell death in AMD: The rationale for targeting Fas. Journal of Clinical Medicine. 2022;**11**(3):7301

[85] Tao Y et al. Necroptosis and Neuroinflammation in retinal degeneration. Frontiers in Neuroscience. 2022;**16**:911430

[86] Yao K et al. RIPK1 in necroptosis and recent progress in related pharmaceutics. Frontiers in Immunology. 2025;**16**:1480027

[87] Murakami Y et al. Programmed necrosis, not apoptosis, is a key mediator of cell loss and DAMP-mediated inflammation in dsRNA-induced retinal degeneration. Cell Death and Differentiation. 2014;**21**(2):270-277

[88] Ou K et al. Marine bromophenols suppressed choroidal neovascularization by targeting HUWE1 through NF-κb signaling pathway. International Journal of Biological Macromolecules. 2024;**257**(Pt 1):128620

[89] Zhang G, Ghosh S. Toll-like receptor-mediated NF-kappaB activation: A phylogenetically conserved paradigm in innate immunity. The Journal of Clinical Investigation. 2001;**107**(1):13-19

[90] Dry AMD: SeaBeLife Achieves Highly Promising Preclinical Efficacy Results for SBL03, without Injections into Eye. 2025. [Internet]. Available from: https://www.seabelife.com/en/dry-amd-seabelife-achieves-highly-promising-preclinical-efficacy-results-for-sbl03-without-injections-into-eye/ [Accessed: May 12, 2025]

[91] Shikamura Y et al. Hydrogel ring for topical drug delivery to the ocular posterior segment. Current Eye Research. 2016;**41**(5):653-661

[92] Ross AE et al. Topical sustained drug delivery to the retina with a drug-eluting contact lens. Biomaterials. 2019;**217**:119285

[93] Navarro-Partida J et al. Lipid-based nanocarriers as topical drug delivery systems for intraocular diseases. Pharmaceutics. 2021;**13**(5):678

[94] Davis BM et al. Topical delivery of Avastin to the posterior segment of the eye in vivo using annexin A5-associated liposomes. Small. 2014;**10**(8):1575-1584

[95] Ying L, Tahara K, Takeuchi H. Drug delivery to the ocular posterior segment using lipid emulsion via eye drop administration: Effect of emulsion formulations and surface modification. International Journal of Pharmaceutics. 2013;**453**(2):329-335

[96] Agarwal P, Rupenthal ID. Non-aqueous formulations in topical ocular drug delivery - a paradigm shift? Advanced Drug Delivery Reviews. 2023;**198**:114867

[97] Kashikar R et al. Ophthalmic nanoemulsion Fingolimod formulation for topical application. Journal of Ocular Pharmacology and Therapeutics. 2024;**40**(8):504-512

[98] Nayak K, Misra M. Triamcinolone Acetonide-loaded PEGylated microemulsion for the posterior segment of eye. ACS Omega. 2020;**5**(14):7928-7939

[99] Vavvas DG et al. Regression of some high-risk features of age-related

macular degeneration (AMD) in patients receiving intensive statin treatment. eBioMedicine. 2016;**5**:198-203

[100] Yadav M et al. Atorvastatin-loaded solid lipid nanoparticles as eye drops: Proposed treatment option for age-related macular degeneration (AMD). Drug Delivery and Translational Research. 2020;**10**:919-944

[101] Liu S et al. Autophagy: Regulator of cell death. Cell Death & Disease. 2023;**14**(10):648

[102] Ambati J, Fowler BJ. Mechanisms of age-related macular degeneration. Neuron. 2012;**75**(1):26-39

[103] Stocchi F, Vacca L, Radicati FG. How to optimize the treatment of early stage Parkinson's disease. Translational Neurodegeneration. 2015;**4**:4

[104] Muto J et al. Highly concentrated trehalose induces prohealing senescence-like state in fibroblasts via CDKN1A/p21. Communications Biology. 2023;**6**(1):13

[105] Ghaem Maralani H et al. Metabolic syndrome and risk of age-related macular degeneration. Retina. 2015;**35**(3):459-466

[106] Adams MK et al. Abdominal obesity and age-related macular degeneration. American Journal of Epidemiology. 2011;**173**(11):1246-1255

[107] Ji PX et al. Improvement in dry age-related macular degeneration with Photobiomodulation. Case Reports in Ophthalmology. 2025;**16**(1):155-162

[108] Hsu SK et al. New insight into the effects of metformin on diabetic retinopathy, aging and cancer: Nonapoptotic cell death, immunosuppression, and effects beyond the AMPK pathway. International Journal of Molecular Sciences. 2021;**22**(17):9453

[109] Han J et al. Metformin suppresses retinal angiogenesis and inflammation in vitro and in vivo. PLoS One. 2018;**13**(3):e0193031

[110] Romdhoniyyah DF et al. Metformin, a potential role in age-related macular degeneration: A systematic review and meta-analysis. Ophthalmology and Therapy. 2021;**10**(2):245-260

[111] Huh MD et al. Potential efficacy of metformin for age-related macular degeneration: A systematic review and meta-analysis. Ophthalmology Science. 2025;**5**(4):100741

Chapter 3

Intergenerational Connections as a Factor in Increasing Age Viability and Reducing Ageism

Karen Samvelovich Bagdasaryan, Larisa Viktorovna Girko, Svetlana Girshevna Gorelik, Alexandra Anatolyevna Melnichenko and Natalya Aleksandrovna Mokicheva

Abstract

In modern society, the demographic process has changed, and the average age of the population is increasing every year. This means that issues related to the viability and quality of life of older people are becoming more relevant. Ageism, which manifests itself in age discrimination, negatively affects the quality of life of older people, their social activity and self-esteem. In addition, in recent decades, intergenerational interaction has become the subject of active research in various fields of knowledge. Research in the field of intergenerational relations and their impact on the viability of older people shows that intergenerational relationships and interaction with other generations contribute to increased self-esteem, the development of life goals and self-realization. Interpersonal relationships, especially within the family, have a significant impact on the viability of older people. Interaction within the family ensures the transfer of experience and values from one generation to another, promotes psychological support and the creation of a positive atmosphere. It is known that a negative view of old age, perception and attitude towards the elderly is formed at an early age, which is reflected in surveys demonstrating ageist stereotypes among the younger generation. Meanwhile, no research has been conducted in Russia on the prevalence of ageism among different age groups, and no attempts have been made to reduce ageism and increase the viability of the older generation by building an active intergenerational dialog and organizing joint events. This "gap" served as the basis for the decision to conduct a study on the impact of intergenerational ties.

Keywords: intergenerational ties, elderly people, vitality, ageism, children

1. Introduction

The problem of social discrimination is a serious and urgent problem of modern society, which is increasingly attracting the attention of researchers. Social discrimination is understood as the restriction of certain human rights on the basis of signs that objectively do not affect their ability to exercise these rights. Age discrimination (ageism) is a type of social discrimination that includes negative attitudes towards people of a certain age group, depriving them of equal rights, etc. It is based on age stereotypes. The term ageism was first used in 1969 by the director of the US National Institute of Aging, Butler. The author understood ageism as negative stereotypes, according to which older people are characterized by senile dementia, rigid attitudes, psychological and social dependence [1]. Let us look at the relationship between age discrimination and psychological well-being in the elderly. The authors Kang and Kim reviewed 13 articles that empirically confirm the negative impact of age discrimination on the psychological well-being of older people [2]. The results of the study showed that an increase in the level of age discrimination is statistically significantly associated with a decrease in psychological well-being among the elderly. In 62% (8 out of 13) of the studies studied, age discrimination was considered as a predictor affecting the psychological well-being of older people using regression analysis. All regressions included control variables such as sociodemographic, socioeconomic, and physical health.

Depression was one of the assessed indicators in 54% (7 out of 13) of the studies. Increased perception or experience of age discrimination was associated with increased symptoms of depression, both stress and anxiety. One study showed that the experience of age discrimination is significantly associated with the prevalence of stress, anxiety disorders, and depression ([3], p. 1458). In another study, it was found that ageism directly affects stress and has an indirect effect on depression through stress [4]. Another author points out that negative age stereotypes are associated with higher levels of depression and loneliness, and low morale. Life satisfaction was assessed in 38% (5 out of 13) of the studies. The results of these studies have shown that perceived ageism and the experience of discrimination are associated with low life satisfaction in the elderly. For example, a study showed that age-based discrimination predicts low life satisfaction among older adults. This corresponds to the results of the study by Ayalon and Ts. There are researchers who have found a negative relationship between perceived discrimination and life satisfaction ([4], p. 156).

Older people face many changes and difficulties that can cause stress and worsen mental health. But there are psychological resources and adaptation strategies that can help older people cope with these problems.

The purpose of our work is to study the level of age discrimination among representatives of different age groups; identification of the role of intergenerational connections in improving the quality of life of the elderly.

2. Research objectives

1. To study the level of knowledge in the field of aging and attitudes towards the older generation in a group of subjects of different ages.

2. To improve the age viability of the older generation through the development of intergenerational ties. We aim to determine how interaction with representatives of other generations affects the emotional well-being, cognitive functions and general perception of the lives of older people.

To achieve this goal, a study was conducted aimed at determining the level of subjectively experienced discrimination by subjects from several age groups—representatives of a group of younger schoolchildren, older schoolchildren and representatives of a group of adults (students of medical universities). The study was conducted over several years (from 2019 to 2023) on the basis of MBOU Gymnasium No. 5 in Belgorod (junior schoolchildren), Bolshetroitskaya Secondary School (high school students), NRU BelSU Medical College (medical students), and the Belgorod Department of Social Protection of the Population, and included three consecutive stages, which were in the nature of a prospective cohort study. A total of 286 people aged 7–19 participated in the study (146 of them were representatives of different age groups to assess the level of intergenerational interaction, 46 younger schoolchildren, 52 elementary school students, 58 students) and the elderly.

Original questionnaires were developed for schoolchildren. The main research method among medical students was the scale of attitudes towards the older generation, developed by Kolpina (a modification of the Kogan scale). These questionnaires and scales were designed to determine the level of subjectively experienced discrimination by subjects representing discriminated groups.

For representatives of the older generation, the research used the method of questioning and interviewing older people. To assess the emotional state, the level of loneliness, and the quality of life of the older generation, standardized questionnaires were used, such as the Psychological General Well–Being Index [5] and the Brief Resilience Scale (BRS). In addition, focus groups were organized for a deeper study of the perception and values of intergenerational relations. The total number of elderly people surveyed was 130 people who were in social institutions and were served at home, as well as elderly people who lead an active social life "Silver Volunteers" aged from 63 to 72 years, of whom 46 received social services in stationary and semi-stationary forms, 84 were pensioners who continue to work. A study was conducted.

At the first stage, the level of knowledge in the field of aging and attitudes towards the older generation were studied (the level of ageism was determined, **Figure 1**) in different age groups using interview methods and questionnaires using original questionnaires.

The first stage was attended by: elementary school students (6–8 years old)—46 people; high school students (15–17 years old)—52 people; Total—98 people [6, 7].

We also decided to assess the level of ageism among medical students (nurses caring for patients); 1st year students (18–19 years old)—58 people;

At the first stage of the study, the viability and quality of life of older age groups were also studied. The study involved: elderly people who are in social service centres, 46 of whom received inpatient and semi-inpatient social services, 84 were pensioners who continue to work.

The following geriatric tools were used: a scale for assessing the Index of General Psychological Well-being; a short scale of age-related vitality; a short questionnaire of quality of life SF-36 (Medical Outcomes Study-Short Form—MOS SF-36, John E. Ware).

Based on the data obtained from the first stages of the study, we have developed a program to increase the age viability of the elderly. The main goal of our program was to reduce the degree of ageism among the younger generation by improving intergenerational ties, as well as increasing the vitality and quality of life of the elderly people participating in the study.

At the second stage of our study, we suggested the following hypothesis: the level of subjectively experienced age discrimination in the group of adolescents and children is at a higher level than in the group of adults. The manifestation of ageism was noted in 76.8% of primary school students.

The manifestation of ageism was detected in 73.7% of high school students (Graph No. 2). Students have a 71.1% level of household ageism (Graph No. 1).

1. Biological determinants of ageism	
IDENTIFICATION OF AGEIST ATTITUDES	
2. Psychosocial determinants of ageism	
The psychological domain	**Own health**
1. Standard educational activities. ⇩ 2. Educational activities on age psychology, development of communication skills, communication with the elderly.	1. Standard educational activities. 2. Educational events on the psychological aspects of ageism, self-development and personal growth. ⇩
Prevention and reduction of age discrimination among the elderly	**Improvement of biological and psychosocial indicators of age-related viability of the elderly**

Figure 1.
Schedule No. 1.

Thus, our hypothesis was confirmed. The level of subjective discrimination in the group of teenagers was higher than in the group of adults. According to the U-Mann–Whitney criterion, differences in the level of discrimination are in the zone of significance (Uemp =41, with $p < 0.01$); therefore, these differences are recognized as statistically significant. The problem of age discrimination, as our research has shown, is relevant, in particular, for adolescents and children (**Figure 2**).

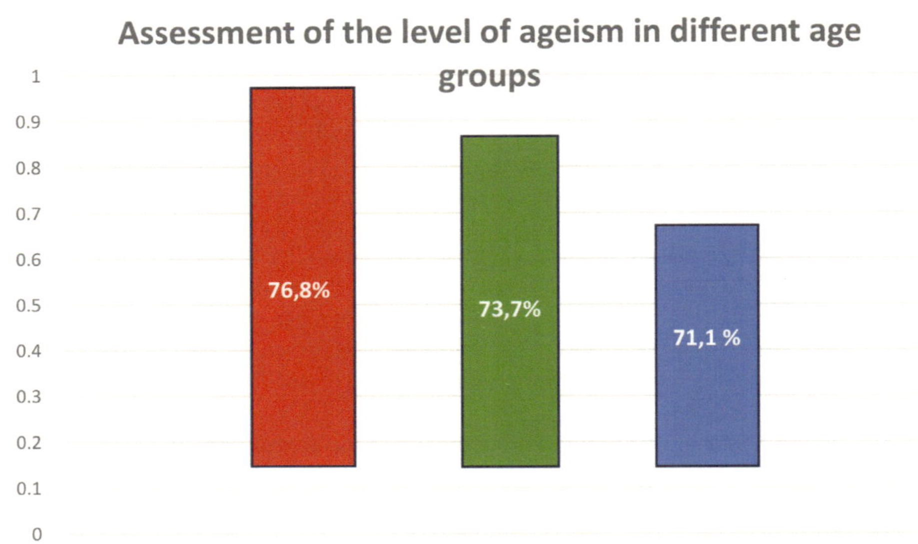

Figure 2.
Schedule No. 2.

At the third stage, we developed and implemented the project "Gerontological education of schoolchildren", which included separate blocks:

1. Project block: Working with younger schoolchildren to develop a program (**Tables 1–4**) for extracurricular activities of younger schoolchildren working with parents and the older generation of younger schoolchildren.

Block 2 of the project is the creation of a volunteer group of different ages and joining the ranks of the "Silver Volunteers of Belgorod region", in which children, together with their parents and older family members, participated in joint activities. The proposed project has been put into practice with an assessment of effectiveness. The effectiveness was determined by: reducing the degree of ageism among schoolchildren and students, improving good manners, improving psychological well-being, vitality and quality of life of the elderly people participating in the project using questionnaires and questionnaires used at the first stage of the study. A total of 300 people aged 7 to 19 took part in the third stage (166 of them were representatives of different age groups, 46 younger schoolchildren, 52 elementary school students, 68 students) and the elderly (134 people) to assess the level of interaction between generations. We conducted a survey of people of different age categories using original questionnaires aimed at determining the level of knowledge in the field of gerontology and geriatrics, the degree of ageism, criteria for the level of education of students and the impact of changing attitudes towards the elderly on the viability of the elderly population after 4 years.

Statistical data processing was carried out using the application software packages Statistica 10 and SAS JMP 11. The statistical significance of the group differences for binary and nominal indicators was determined using the Pearson Chi-square test. The level of statistical significance was fixed at 0.05.

№	Topic	Content	Methods and forms
1	What is age?	The concepts of childhood, adulthood and old age.	Interactive conversation, working with a calendar of ages, a person's life line.
2	How does a person change with age?	Physical and emotional changes.	The game "Portrait at different ages".
3	Who are the elderly?	A conversation about grandparents and their roles.	Painting "My grandmother/grandfather."
4	An elderly man is interesting!	Stories and hobbies of the elderly, their grandparents.	A story or a meeting with elderly volunteers. Holiday Fair.
5	Stereotypes about old age.	What is bias, and why old age is not scary.	Comparative analysis of images/persistent stereotypes about old age in children, the game "Myth and Truth".
6	How are older people like children?	Emotions, needs, care.	Game "Guess by the expression on his face." Drawings, stories, stories: how children resemble their grandparents.
7	Why respect the elderly?	Family values, traditions.	Creative task "Tree of respect".
8	The result of the module: "Me and my elders"	An exhibition of drawings, mini-stories.	Project format, presentation, creation of a "Family tree"

Table 1.
Objective: To form children's understanding of old age as a natural and respected stage of life.

№	Topic	Content	Methods and forms
9	What is health?	Introduction to the concept of physical and psycho-emotional health.	"Health portfolio" (modeling, application).
10	Why does health begin in childhood?	Principles of a healthy lifestyle.	Group work: we collect the "right day", an analysis of mandatory routine actions to preserve health.
11	Healthy lifestyle and aging.	How what we do today affects the future.	Cartoons with discussion.
12	Move like a grandmother!	Exercises that are useful for all ages.	Joint charging (video or live example), filling out checklists for a month/3/9 about joint exercise with elderly relatives.
13	Nutrition and age.	Healthy food for children and the elderly.	The game "Collect a plate of health".
14	Sleep, water, sun—health is all around.	Habits that promote health.	Quest is a healthy lifestyle game.
15	Emotions and health.	How mood affects well-being.	Exercise "Mood color". Filling out a checklist for a month/3/9 about your mood (in class, at home)
16	Illness and care.	Why do the elderly get sick more often and how can we help them.	Role-playing game: "I'm an assistant."
17	Memory, attention, and brain training.	Development of cognitive functions.	Memory and attention games.
18	The result of the module: "How to be healthy all your life"	Presentation of the book "How to become a healthy old man."	Teamwork.

Table 2.
Objective: To form the belief that one's own health since childhood influences active and successful aging in the future.

№	Topic	Content	Methods and forms
19	What is friendship between generations?	Different interests, but common communication.	Reading works about the importance of passing on the experience of the older generation to the younger.
20	What do our elders teach us?	Wisdom, experience, traditions.	Interactive: "Advice from Grandma." Children collect advice from their older relatives and read it to the class.
21	Visiting my grandmother.	Ethics of behaviour, help.	Creating a memo "How to be a kind grandson."
22	Good deeds for the elders.	Real ways to help.	Project: "I help my grandmother around the house."
23	Joint holidays	Why it's important to celebrate holidays together.	Preparation of congratulations.
24	In the world of hobbies	Hobbies of the older and younger ones.	A master class from grandma/grandpa.
25	A letter to the grandson of the future	Wishes for yourself in old age.	A personality-oriented task.

№	Topic	Content	Methods and forms
26	A small volunteer	A conversation about help and support.	The game situation is "I am a volunteer".
27	The result of the module: "Me and my older friends"	A flash mob, a social day, a celebration for their grandparents, a guest visit with a festive concert at a nursing home, etc.	

Table 3.
Objective: To develop children's intergenerational skills and an understanding of the importance of communicating with elders.

№	Topic	Content	Methods and forms
28	Old age is about the future	We think: "What will I be like in my old age?"	Drawings of "Me at 80".
29	I choose to be healthy.	We model our lives: food, movement, good deeds.	The game "The Way of health".
30	What would a world like where elders are respected be like?	The values of kindness and mutual assistance.	Group fairy tale, performance, creation of a plasticine city
31	Everyone ages differently.	The diversity of old age.	Comparative analysis "Who ages how?" using the example of people, animals, and plants.
32	What can I do for the elders?	Reflection.	Circle of care: a practical task. A record of good deeds and help for older people.
33	Me and my health	The results of personal growth.	Self-assessment of habits.
34	A gift for an elderly friend	Preparation of a collective gift / postcard.	Creative workshop.
35	The Feast of Goodness	A joint event with the invitation of the elderly.	Concert, exhibition of works, fair.
36	Bottom line: "I am a friend of the elders, I am a friend of myself in the future"	Summing up, discussions.	A solemn lesson.

Table 4.
Goal: To create an image of the future in children, in which active aging is possible due to the efforts already being made.

3. Conclusions

Ageism is defined as negative stereotypes about older people that lead to discrimination, segregation, and neglect [8]. For example, older people who adhere to and internalize negative age stereotypes and attitudes decrease cognitive and physical activity. There is general agreement in our rapidly aging societies that ageism should be combated in order to promote healthier aging and better integration of older people into social activities. Generational Engagement Programs (PVP) are an effective tool for combating ageism, contributing to the mutual enrichment of experience and knowledge between different age groups, as well as these programs improve the viability of older people, and reduce depression.

Negative views and attitudes towards the elderly can begin at an early age. When school-age children are asked what they think about the elderly, they often reveal negative views and ageist stereotypes [6, 7].

The study confirmed the high prevalence of ageism and gerontological stereotypes among schoolchildren, mostly in the lower grades 76.8%. When studying the attitude of younger schoolchildren to old age, the following data were obtained: that slightly less than half (44.0%) believe that living in old age is hard, difficult and the life of an elderly person is very bad. A total of 39.2% of children believe that life is sad in old age; 22.4% of children think the life of an elderly person is interesting and fun; 9.6% think it is respected. Perhaps such answers are related to children's feelings that during this period of life people only relax and do what they love.

When the children were asked to write five words about how they perceive the elderly, it turned out that 21.1% consider them wise, 12.3% kind. But 17.5% believe that older people constantly need help, 9.6% believe that older people are constantly sick. A total of 15.8% of younger students noted that it is very difficult for them to communicate with older people and older people, including their grandparents, do not understand them. The connection of ageist attitudes with a number of factors has been revealed. Firstly, the lack of live communication with the elderly contributes to the persistence of prejudice. Respondents who do not live with older relatives are less aware of their health status and are less likely to participate in helping them, which indicates a more pronounced disregard for the needs of the elderly. On the contrary, permanent cohabitation with elderly relatives turns out to be a factor that reduces the tendency to ageism: there is a more positive perception of the older generation. Secondly, there are psychological reasons: the respondents themselves.

Author details

Karen Samvelovich Bagdasaryan[1], Larisa Viktorovna Girko[1], Svetlana Girshevna Gorelik[2], Alexandra Anatolyevna Melnichenko[1*] and Natalya Aleksandrovna Mokicheva[3]

1 Department of Gerontology and Geriatrics of the Medical Institute of the Belgorod State National Research University, Belgorod, Russia

2 Department of Health Organization and Public Health, Federal State Autonomous Educational Institution of Higher Education "Belgorod State National Research University", Belgorod, Russia

3 Medical Sciences, Department of Social Work, Economics, and Bioethics, Yaroslavl State Medical University, Yaroslavl, Russia

*Address all correspondence to: sanka_melnichenk@mail.ru

References

[1] Makarova EY. International scientific and practical conference "evolution, progress and modernization". Age Discrimination Experienced by Representatives of Different Age Groups. Collection of Scientific Papers based on the Materials of the International Scientific and Practical Conference of Students, Magisters and Postgraduate Students. Professional Science NGO; 2017. pp. 287-292

[2] Akhtyan AG, Anikeeva OA, Sizikova VV, Shimanovskaya YV, Starovoytova LI, Medvedeva GP, et al. Information literacy of older people: Social aspects of the problem. International Journal of Civil Engineering and Technology. 2018;**9**(11):1789-1799

[3] Lyons A, Alba B, Heywood W, Fileborn B, Minichiello V, Barrett C, et al. Experiences of ageism and the mental health of older adults. Aging & Mental Health. 2018;**22**(11):1456-1464. DOI: 10.1080/13607863.2017.1364347

[4] Defining intergenerational practice [Electronic resource] II Access mode. Available from: http://www.volstudy.ac.uk/Intergen/IntergenerationalDefined.litml

[5] Gorelik SG, Ilnitsky AN, Proshchaev KI, Bogat SV. Database Methodological Guide "Specialized Geriatric Examination". Certificate No. 2015620486, Registration Date. 16.03.2015

[6] Melnichenko AA, Gorelik SG. Ageism as a problem of the younger generation. Cardiovascular Therapy and Prevention. 2023;**22**(S3):68-70

[7] Melnichenko AA, Gorelik SG. Studying the level of gerontological knowledge of primary school students. Modern Problems of Healthcare and Medical Statistics. 2023;**2**:337-347

[8] Afanasyeva TS. Gerontophobia and ageism as dangers for children and youth in a post-industrial society. In: Deviantology of Parenthood. Collection of Scientific Papers; 2016

Chapter 4

Water-Based Wellness: Unlocking Physical Resilience and Functional Longevity in Ageing Population

Aryan Shukla

Abstract

As the global population ages, a pressing gap emerges between lifespan and health span marked by chronic degeneration, immobility, and psychosocial decline. Traditional geriatric care often fails to address the complex interplay of physical, emotional, and cognitive wellness. This chapter explores hydrotherapy as a transformative, science-backed intervention in geriatric care. Drawing from physiology, neuroscience, and rehabilitation medicine, it outlines how water-based therapy supports function preservation, joint health, balance, and cardiovascular safety while also reducing anxiety, isolation, and fear of falls. With principles grounded in buoyancy, thermodynamics, and hydrostatic pressure, hydrotherapy creates a joint-friendly environment that fosters movement without strain. The chapter also reviews various modalities including warm water therapy, aquatic tai chi, contrast baths, and underwater treadmill training, comparing their outcomes with land-based therapies. Practical models for integrating hydrotherapy into elderly routines are also presented, along with strategies to overcome barriers like infrastructure, cost, and professional availability. By linking clinical evidence with real-world applications, this text presents hydrotherapy not just as a rehabilitative tool but as an essential component of preventive strategy that enhances autonomy, dignity, and long-term well-being in older adults.

Keywords: geriatric wellness, low-impact exercises, hydrotherapy, healthy ageing, fall prevention

1. Introduction

The world is undergoing a demographic shift, with people over 60 years expected to outnumber those under 15 for the first time in history by 2050 [1]. This transition brings with it an urgent concern: how do we ensure quality of life, not just longevity? Ageing is inherently accompanied by chronic degenerative processes like decreased joint flexibility, reduced vascularity, generalised sarcopenia and neurological decline [2]. These factors contribute to disability associated with falls, reduced functional independence, and increased healthcare dependency among the elderly. Amidst this, we face a pressing "wellness gap," the growing division between lifespan and health-span. While advances in medicine have extended human life expectancy, they have not proportionately improved the years lived in good health. This paradox presents both a clinical challenge and an opportunity for how we maintain function, mobility, and dignity as people age. Hydrotherapy, a therapeutic approach involving the use of water for pain relief and treatment, is emerging as a promising solution. By harnessing the principles of buoyancy, resistance, hydrostatic pressure, and temperature, hydrotherapy allows ageing individuals to engage in functional activity without the strain imposed by gravity [3]. The buoyancy of water reduces joint load, enabling movement even in individuals with osteoarthritis or frailty. Hydrostatic pressure improves venous return and circulation, while warm water supports muscle relaxation and pain modulation [4]. Multiple randomised controlled trials and meta-analyses support the effectiveness of hydrotherapy, like Vivas et al. [5] found that aquatic therapy significantly improved balance and reduced the fear of falling in community-dwelling older adults. Another study by Noh et al. [6] highlighted improved gait patterns and confidence among stroke patients receiving aquatic therapy, illustrating its neurological benefits. Psychologically, hydrotherapy has also been shown to reduce symptoms of anxiety and depression and to increase motivation for physical activity among the elderly [7]. These findings align with the biopsychosocial model of ageing, emphasising the interdependence of mind and body in therapeutic outcomes. Incorporating hydrotherapy into ageing care offers a regenerative model—one that not only rehabilitates but revitalises. It bridges the gap between ageing and wellness by restoring function, dignity, and autonomy. As healthcare systems grapple with ageing populations, hydrotherapy represents an integrative, evidence-based tool for future-ready rehabilitation.

A compelling example of this integrative potential can be found in the National Health Service (NHS) in the United Kingdom, where community hydrotherapy programmes are being implemented for elderly patients with osteoarthritis, Parkinson's disease, and post-stroke impairments. In these programmes, patients report not only improvements in functional independence and balance but also reductions in pain perception and fear of falling [5, 7]. This model reflects the evolving approach in geriatric rehabilitation, which increasingly prioritises holistic, person-centred care. It emphasises functional improvement rather than merely managing symptoms and promotes proactive maintenance instead of reactive crisis intervention. However, the development and implementation of such comprehensive care systems remain limited. These progressive shifts are primarily observed in well-developed regions and advanced healthcare settings. The true challenge lies in underserved and under-resourced areas, where ageing populations continue to struggle for basic functional mobility and pain-free quality of life.

2. Geriatric wellness: The emerging crisis

The emerging crisis is not merely about longevity but the capacity to live well in advanced age. Ageing populations are exerting tremendous pressure on healthcare systems worldwide. While life expectancy has increased substantially, this has not been matched by a proportional rise in "Health-Adjusted Life Expectancy" (HALE)—a metric that quantifies years lived without disability [8]. In many countries, particularly those with ageing societies like Japan, Italy, and Germany, the final decades of life are increasingly characterised by comorbidities, frailty, cognitive decline, and loss of autonomy. This rising burden is especially challenging for healthcare economies. For instance, in the United States, over 80% of older adults live with at least one chronic condition, such as arthritis, hypertension, diabetes, or heart disease, and more than 60% live with two or more [9]. The financial cost of treating chronic illnesses in the elderly consumes a significant share of national healthcare budgets. Moreover, these "Geriatric syndromes" often lead to repeated hospitalisations, long-term medication use and a growing dependence on social and caregiver support systems, thereby intensifying economic and societal strain. The concept of these syndromes captures a set of multifactorial conditions that are not tied to a single disease process but have shared risk factors and significant impacts on functionality and quality of life. These include frailty, falls, urinary incontinence, cognitive impairment, pressure ulcers, and delirium [10]. Such syndromes often interact in complex ways, leading to a cascade of functional deterioration and reduced resilience in older adults. For example, frailty, a clinical syndrome characterised by unintentional weight loss, weakness, exhaustion, slow walking speed, and low physical activity, affects approximately 10–15% of community-dwelling older adults [11]. Frail individuals are more susceptible to hospitalisation, disability, and mortality, even after minor stressors like a cold or a brief period of immobility. Similarly, sarcopenia and osteoporosis lead to impaired mobility and an increased risk of falls, which are the leading cause of injury-related deaths in adults over 65 [12]. These physical declines are often compounded by cognitive syndromes such as mild cognitive impairment or dementia, creating a multidimensional burden on the individual and their support systems.

One of the central paradoxes in modern ageing is the widening gap between longevity and quality of life. Medical advancements have significantly prolonged human lifespan, but these extra years are frequently accompanied by a progressive decline in autonomy, purpose, and engagement. This paradox is stark: while people are living longer, they are not necessarily living better. The concept of "compression of morbidity," proposed by Fries [13], suggests that with effective preventive strategies, the period of disability and illness before death can be shortened, thereby enhancing the quality of life even as people live longer. However, in reality, many older adults experience an "expansion of morbidity," where chronic diseases and disabilities extend over

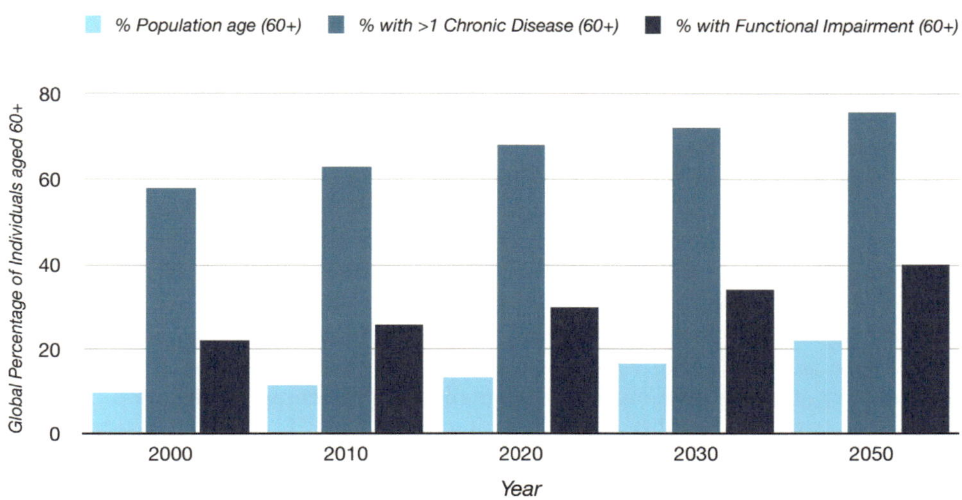

Figure 1.
The above data illustrates the rising global burden of ageing, chronic disease prevalence and functional decline in older adults from 2000 to projected levels in 2050 [1, 15–17].

many years. The misalignment between years lived and years lived well is not only a medical concern but a philosophical and ethical one. Increasing evidence shows that psychosocial factors—such as loneliness, loss of purpose, and social isolation—have a measurable impact on health outcomes, often equating in significance to traditional risk factors like smoking and obesity [14]. Thus, the solution lies not merely in adding years to life but in adding life to years. A function-oriented model of ageing must prioritise mobility, independence, cognitive vitality, and social participation. The WHO's Decade of Healthy Ageing (2021–2030) [1] emphasises intrinsic capacity: the composite of all the physical and mental capacities an individual can draw on and functional ability as central goals for health systems (**Figure 1**).

As the geriatric wellness crisis looms larger, it is no longer sufficient to view ageing as a medical condition. It is a complex life stage requiring a multidisciplinary approach that spans biology, behaviour, environment, and policy. The goal should not be simply to extend life but to ensure that those additional years are meaningful, active, and dignified.

3. Functional ageing under pressure: Systemic and psychosocial barriers

Ageing is intrinsically associated with a progressive deterioration of musculoskeletal integrity, which critically undermines functional independence in the elderly. Among the most prominent manifestations of this decline is sarcopenia, a condition marked by the gradual and debilitating loss of skeletal muscle mass, strength, and endurance. This multifactorial syndrome arises through complex physiological processes that converge to weaken the neuromuscular system. The primary physiological precursor responsible for initiating the cascade is neuromuscular degradation, where ageing-associated functional decline and reduced muscle force output lead to a marked reduction in both the quantity and functionality of α-motor neurons. This decline impairs motor unit recruitment and induces muscle fibre denervation and subsequent atrophy, particularly of fast-twitch fibres, resulting in diminished coordination, slower reflexes, and increased susceptibility to falls [18]. Additionally, age-related hormonal alterations further exacerbate sarcopenia. A decline in anabolic hormones such as testosterone, growth hormone (GH), and insulin-like growth factor-1 (IGF-1) impairs protein synthesis pathways that are essential for muscle hypertrophy and regeneration. The reduction in IGF-1 in particular limits the activation of satellite cells which are crucial for muscle repair, thus weakening the body's adaptive response to muscular stress or injury [19]. Simultaneously, mitochondrial dysfunction plays a pivotal role in accelerating muscular degradation. With ageing, mitochondria exhibit decreased oxidative phosphorylation efficiency and increased production of reactive oxygen species (ROS), leading to ATP insufficiency and elevated oxidative damage within muscle fibres. This imbalance disrupts cellular homeostasis and induces apoptotic signalling, which promotes muscle cell death and further amplifies sarcopenic progression [20]. Together, these interlinked mechanisms create a physiological cascade that not only erodes muscle performance but also compromises mobility, resilience to stress, and quality of life in ageing individuals (**Figure 2**). Understanding these mechanisms underscores the importance of early intervention strategies targeting neuromuscular health, hormonal balance, and mitochondrial function in order to preserve functional longevity and reduce dependency in the elderly.

In parallel with muscular decline, ageing also brings about progressive joint dysfunction, with osteoarthritis (OA) emerging as one of the most common and

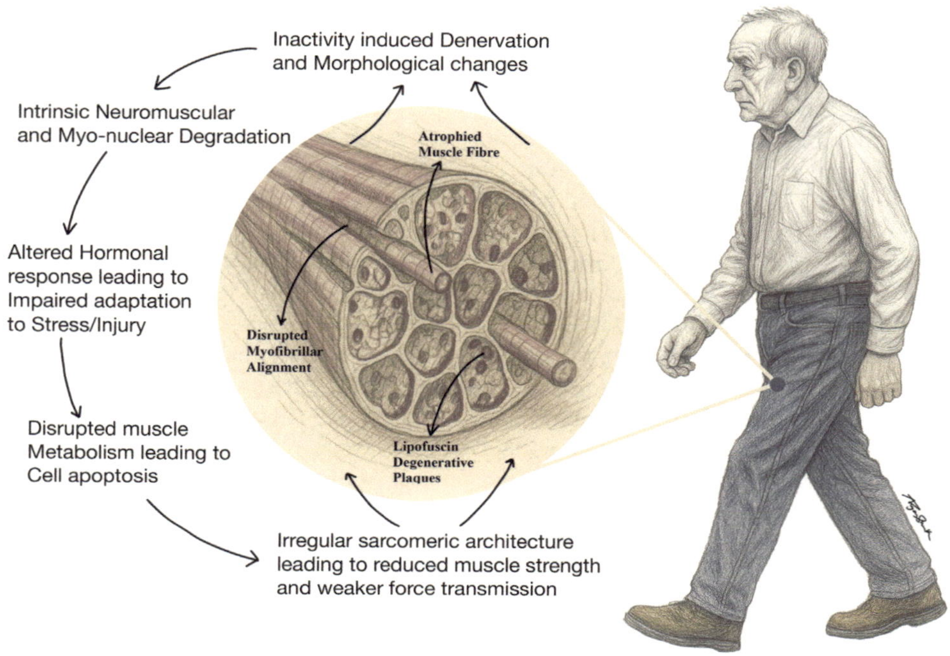

Figure 2.
The sarcopenic cascade—a progressive degeneration leading to muscle weakness and impaired functional capacity [18, 20].

debilitating conditions affecting older adults. The pathogenesis of OA is primarily driven by the degradation of articular cartilage, which serves as a shock-absorbing surface within joints. With advancing age, chondrocytes, the specialised cells that maintain the volume of cartilage, exhibit reduced autophagic activity, impairing their ability to clear damaged cellular components. Simultaneously, these ageing cells up-regulate the production of matrix metalloproteinases (MMPs) and other catabolic enzymes, leading to accelerated extracellular matrix breakdown and a consequent loss of chondral integrity. These changes result in a narrowing of the intra-articular space with extra-articular irritation and pain, leading to a decreased range of motion [21]. Beyond the cartilage, subchondral bone - the layer of bone just beneath the cartilage, also undergoes age-related remodelling impairments. Ageing disturbs the balance between bone resorption and formation, leading to increased bone fragility, microfractures, and structural instability across load-bearing articular surfaces of the major joints such as hips and knees. This compromised support accelerates the degenerative cycle, further weakening joint mechanics and function. The combined effects of musculoskeletal decline and age-associated sensory deterioration including reduced visual acuity, impaired proprioception, and progressive vestibular dysfunction substantially heighten the risk of falls in older adults. These deficits compromise spatial awareness and dynamic balance, making individuals more prone to tripping, misstepping, or experiencing disorientation, all of which directly impair postural stability and coordination. As a result, comprehensive fall prevention strategies become a necessity in geriatric care.

While physical deterioration is a hallmark of ageing, the psychosocial challenges that accompany later life stages often remain un recognised and untreated, despite their profound impact on overall health and functional independence. Social isolation is common among older adults due to retirement, bereavement, reduced mobility, or institutionalisation, which is more than a social concern with deep physiological and neurological repercussions. Studies demonstrate that social disconnectedness is associated with accelerated cognitive decline, particularly due to the lack of mental and emotional stimulation, which reduces synaptic activity and neuroplasticity, thus increasing the risk of dementia [22]. Moreover, loneliness has been correlated with elevated levels of cortisol and inflammatory cytokines such as interleukin-6 (IL-6) and C-reactive protein (CRP), contributing to hypertension and cardiovascular morbidity. In parallel, depression and anxiety are prevalent yet frequently underdiagnosed in elderly populations. This under-diagnosis often results from overlapping symptoms with other medical conditions and the false assumption that low mood is a normal aspect of ageing. Biologically, ageing affects neurotransmitter systems, notably serotonin and dopamine, making older individuals more susceptible to mood disorders. Additionally, life transitions such as loss of social roles, economic insecurity, and chronic illness further amplify psychological distress. According to a recent meta-analysis, global prevalence rates of depression and anxiety in older adults are approximately 19.2% and 16.5%, respectively [23], highlighting the urgent need for systematic screening and early psychological intervention.

3.1 The invisible burden of systemic barriers undermining geriatric health

The healthcare system often struggles to accommodate the layered, multidimensional needs of the ageing population. A key issue is the underdiagnosis and under-treatment of serious conditions due to atypical presentations. For instance, myocardial infarction in the elderly may occur without chest pain, and infections may present without classic febrile responses due to blunted immune reactivity [24]. Ageism in clinical decision-making leads to the erroneous belief that symptoms are part of “natural ageing,” resulting in therapeutic nihilism and delayed interventions. Furthermore, communication gaps arising from sensory deficits such as hearing loss or cognitive impairments hinder proper history-taking, treatment adherence, and follow-up care. Compounding this, caregiver strain is a critical but frequently neglected domain. Caregivers, particularly family members, face intense emotional and psychological burdens, including guilt, anxiety, and burnout, especially when caring for individuals with dementia or complex disabilities [25]. The physical demands of caregiving can result in musculoskeletal injuries, while financial stress arises from reduced employment opportunities, lack of insurance support, and minimal access to respite care. In low- and middle-income regions, where geriatric infrastructure is sparse, these challenges are significantly magnified. Fragmented healthcare systems, insufficient training for home-based care, and limited access to mental health services create a persistent cycle of unmet needs, accelerating functional decline and leading to caregiver exhaustion. As a result, the combined impact of physiological, psychosocial, and systemic challenges significantly undermines geriatric care and functional longevity across multiple domains, particularly beyond the early stages of ageing (**Table 1**). Another critical and often underestimated contributor is polypharmacy, commonly defined as the use of five or more medications. It is a growing concern in geriatric care, with prevalence rates exceeding 40%, as older adults are frequently prescribed multiple medications for chronic conditions [26]. Many of these drugs, including antihypertensives, sedatives, and antidepressants, are associated with side effects like dizziness, orthostatic hypotension, and delayed

Sr. no.	Domain	Challenges
(1)	Physical decline	Sarcopenia
		Joint dysfunction and osteoarthritis
		Increased risk of falls
(2)	Neuromuscular function	Mitochondrial dysfunction
		Motor neuron loss and denervation
		Central motor control deficits
(3)	Psychosocial limitations	Social isolation
		Depression and anxiety
(4)	Systemic healthcare issues	Under-diagnosis of conditions
		Under-treatment and delayed interventions
		Caregiver but put and strain

Table 1.
Key physiological, psychosocial, and systemic challenges affecting geriatric care and functional longevity [18, 21, 23, 25].

reaction time, which directly impair balance and coordination. While necessary for managing multiple chronic conditions, polypharmacy increases the risk of adverse drug events (ADEs) that directly impair physical and cognitive function. Medications such as antihypertensives can cause orthostatic hypotension, sedatives can lead to drowsiness and impaired motor coordination, and antidepressants may provoke dizziness and delayed reaction times—all of which elevate the likelihood of falls [27, 28]. Furthermore, drug-drug interactions (DDI) and age-related changes in pharmacokinetics and pharmacodynamics compound these risks. Therefore, regular medication reviews and deprescribing protocols should be integral to holistic fall prevention strategies in geriatric rehabilitation.

4. Models and strategies for promoting geriatric wellness

Promoting geriatric wellness is a multifaceted endeavour that necessitates a comprehensive understanding of ageing processes and the implementation of holistic strategies. This discussion delves into three pivotal components: the World Health Organisation's (WHO) frameworks for healthy ageing, multidimensional and biopsychosocial models, and the integral roles of exercise, socialisation, and engagement.

4.1 WHO frameworks for healthy ageing

The WHO has been at the forefront of advocating for healthy ageing, emphasising the importance of maintaining the functional ability to ensure well-being in older age. Their approach is encapsulated in the "Decade of Healthy Ageing (2021–2030)," a global initiative aimed at improving the lives of older people, their families, and communities [1]. Central to this framework is the concept of "functional ability," which refers to the health-related attributes that enable people to be and do what they value. This encompasses the capacity to meet basic needs, learn and make decisions, be mobile, build and maintain relationships, and contribute to society [15]. The WHO's approach underscores the need for action across multiple sectors, including health, education, labour, and social protection, to create environments that support healthy ageing. This holistic perspective recognises that ageing is not solely a health issue but is influenced by a myriad of social and environmental factors.

4.2 Multidimensional and biopsychosocial models

Understanding ageing through a multidimensional and biopsychosocial lens is essential for constructing comprehensive strategies that truly promote geriatric wellness. These models help us move beyond a disease-centric perspective to one that acknowledges the complexity and diversity of ageing experiences across individuals. The biopsychosocial model, first introduced by George Engel in 1977, emphasises that health outcomes are shaped not solely by biological mechanisms but also by psychological states (such as cognition, emotion, and motivation) and social environments (including relationships, support systems, and socioeconomic status) [29]. In geriatric care, this model provides a valuable framework for addressing both the visible and hidden aspects of ageing. For example, an elderly patient with osteoarthritis may also be experiencing depression, loneliness, and financial strain—factors that amplify pain perception, reduce adherence to treatment and compromise quality of life. Complementing this, the multidimensional model of ageing outlines key domains influencing overall well-being: physical function, cognitive health, emotional status, social engagement, functional independence, and environmental conditions [30]. This model is widely used in geriatric assessments such as the Comprehensive Geriatric Assessment (CGA), which helps clinicians evaluate older adults beyond their primary diagnosis, incorporating aspects like nutrition, mental status, mobility, and living situation to form personalised interventions [31]. These frameworks collectively challenge the reductionist notion that successful ageing is merely the absence of disease. Instead, they propose that optimal ageing includes maintaining autonomy, participating in meaningful social roles, and adapting positively to age-related changes. This aligns with Rowe and Kahn's model of successful ageing, which identifies three main components: a low probability of disease, high physical and cognitive functioning, and active engagement with life [32]. Empirical support for the biopsychosocial model continues to grow. A study comparing older adults in Pakistan and Canada found that variables such as health status, self-efficacy, social support, and self-esteem significantly influenced perceived quality of life, regardless of geographical or cultural differences [33]. These findings underscore that biopsychosocial factors are universally relevant and can guide ageing-related policy and care planning globally. Importantly, the models also acknowledge the reciprocal nature of these domains. Social isolation, for example, may reduce motivation for self-care, which in turn exacerbates health decline and increases dependency. Conversely, strong social ties and a sense of purpose can improve adherence to medical treatments, boost immune function, and mitigate stress-related damage [34]. Furthermore, incorporating psychological resilience—defined as the capacity to recover from stress or adversity—has shown protective effects in geriatric populations.

Older adults with higher resilience tend to exhibit better emotional regulation, reduced frailty, and improved cognitive outcomes, even when facing chronic illness or disability [35]. Together, the biopsychosocial and multidimensional models serve as indispensable tools for ageing research and practice. They support the idea that effective geriatric care must not only address medical issues but also nurture psychological health and create supportive environments that empower the elderly to live with dignity, purpose, and independence.

4.3 Role of exercise, socialisation, and engagement in geriatric wellness

Physical activity is widely recognised as a foundational component of healthy ageing, offering profound physiological, cognitive, and psychosocial benefits. Regular physical exercise contributes to the preservation of skeletal muscle mass, enhances neuromuscular coordination, and maintains cardiovascular efficiency—factors that are critical for mobility, fall prevention, and independence in older adults [36, 37]. Resistance and balance training, in particular, have been shown to reduce the risk of sarcopenia and frailty, conditions commonly associated with ageing and linked to increased morbidity and mortality [2]. Aerobic activities, such as walking, cycling, and swimming, have consistently been associated with reduced incidence of non-communicable diseases including type 2 diabetes, hypertension, stroke, and cardiovascular disease [38]. Exercise is also neuroprotective as physical activity stimulates the release of neurotrophic factors such as brain-derived neurotrophic factor (BDNF), which supports neurogenesis, synaptic plasticity, and cognitive preservation in ageing populations [39]. Beyond these physiological benefits, exercise plays a central role in enhancing psychological health. Regular movement has been shown to reduce symptoms of depression and anxiety by modulating neurotransmitter function and improving sleep quality [40]. Critically, many forms of physical activity—particularly group-based programmes—naturally foster social interaction, which is equally important for geriatric wellness. Engaging in activities like community walking groups, yoga classes, or recreational sports provides not only motivation for sustained participation but also strengthens a sense of belonging, combats loneliness, and improves emotional well-being [41, 42].

Socialisation, as a determinant of healthy ageing, extends beyond exercise. According to the activity theory of ageing, older adults achieve greater life satisfaction and better functional outcomes when they remain socially engaged in roles that provide meaning and stimulation [43]. Active participation in social activities such as religious gatherings, hobby clubs, or cultural events contributes to enhanced mood, cognitive resilience, and even decreased mortality risk [14, 44]. Community engagement further amplifies these benefits by offering older adults a sense of agency and purpose. Volunteering, participating in civic activities, or mentoring younger generations allows individuals to maintain a meaningful identity and remain integrated in societal structures. Data from the National Health and Aging Trends Study (NHATS) demonstrate that older adults who regularly engage in physical and social activities report higher levels of psychological well-being, reduced functional decline, and slower cognitive deterioration [45]. In sum, integrating physical activity with meaningful social interaction and community participation is essential for promoting holistic wellness among older adults. These lifestyle behaviours not only mitigate the risks associated with physiological ageing but also foster emotional resilience, cognitive health, and a sense of purpose, all of which are crucial for maintaining the quality of life in later years.

5. Principles of hydrotherapy: Scientific basis and application in geriatric care

Hydrotherapy is known as a form of therapy which refers to the clinical application of water in various temperatures, states (liquid, steam, or ice), and delivery methods (immersion, compresses, jets, etc.) to treat a range of pathological conditions by utilising its mechanical and thermal effects. It has become increasingly recognised in modern rehabilitation settings for its diverse, evidence-backed physiological and psychological benefits. Particularly in geriatric populations, hydrotherapy represents a multidimensional therapeutic tool that not only targets biomechanical impairments but also addresses underlying circulatory, neurological, and psychosocial deficits often neglected in conventional land-based rehabilitation approaches. As individuals age, they encounter a progressive decline across various physiological systems. In such cases, hydrotherapy provides a safe, supportive, and low-impact environment that mitigates these limitations while maximising functional physiological gains (**Table 2**).

Sr. no.	Physiological system	Adaptation	Clinical outcome
(1)	Musculoskeletal system	Improved density of type 2a muscle fibres	Enhanced response ability of the soft tissues under load resulting in better movement quality.
		Enhanced mitochondrial volume	
		Improved joint play	
(2)	Neuromuscular system	Enhanced firing of alpha motor neurons	Improved response time with better sense of stability and postural control while in motion or change of direction.
		Improved efferent conductivity of neurons	
		Enhanced excitability of the central motor pools	
(3)	Cardiovascular system	Improved cardiac dynamics and symmetry	Improved coherence between physiological load and associated cardiac changes.
		Improved coronary circulatory efficiency	
(4)	Pulmonary system	Improved alveolar sensitivity	Improved pulmonary endurance and functional capacity resulting in enhanced locomotory ability
		Improved parenchymal micro circulation	
(5)	Endocrine system	Improved insulin sensitivity	Improved glycemic control with reduction in cardiovascular risk.
		Improved hormonal associated mechanical gains	
(6)	Immune system	Improved lymphatic drainage and circulation	Better chemical response of the body towards exercise which enhances exercise related sensitivity of the body and long-term adaptations.
		Reduction in production of inflammatory markers	
		Decreased low grade inflammation across joints	

Table 2.
System-specific physiological adaptations induced by hydrotherapy in geriatric individuals [3].

5.1 Thermodynamic effects of hydrotherapy

The thermodynamic properties of water—specifically its temperature regulation capacity—are fundamental to hydrotherapy's therapeutic value, particularly in geriatric populations. Water can be precisely temperature-controlled, making it an ideal medium for delivering targeted thermal interventions, whether to relax muscles, reduce inflammation, modulate neural activity, or enhance circulation [46].

5.1.1 Warm water immersion (33–36°C)

Warm water therapy is most commonly used in rehabilitation settings for elderly patients. Immersion in water at thermoneutral to mildly warm temperatures (33–36°C) offers several physiological and therapeutic benefits.

5.1.1.1 Vasodilation and improved peripheral circulation

Heat causes vasodilation of cutaneous and muscular blood vessels, increasing blood flow to peripheral tissues. This enhances oxygen delivery and waste product removal, promoting tissue healing and reducing stiffness in age-compromised musculoskeletal structures [47]. This is particularly beneficial in elderly patients with peripheral artery disease, diabetes-related microvascular issues, or chronic cold extremities.

5.1.1.2 Reduction in muscle tone and joint stiffness

Warmth helps decrease alpha motor neuron excitability, leading to a reduction in muscle tone and spasm—a key benefit for patients suffering from post-stroke spasticity or Parkinsonian rigidity [3]. Moreover, increased elasticity of connective tissue at elevated temperatures improves joint mobility and range of motion, which is critical in conditions such as osteoarthritis, frozen shoulder, or ankylosing spondylitis common in older adults.

5.1.1.3 Pain modulation

The application of heat in hydrotherapy activates thermo receptors that override nociceptive input *via* the gate control theory of pain. This results in immediate analgesic effects without pharmacological side effects, making it a preferred option in geriatric patients who often have polypharmacy concerns or contraindications for NSAIDs.

5.1.1.4 Facilitation of gentle exercise

When combined with the effects of buoyancy and hydrostatic pressure, warm water further allows elderly individuals with limited mobility to perform exercises that may be too painful or difficult on land. The warmth reduces joint friction, promoting safe movement initiation and prolonged activity tolerance, especially in frail or deconditioned elderly individuals.

5.1.1.5 Improved sleep and autonomic nervous regulation

Research indicates that warm water immersion has a parasympathetic-dominant effect, reducing sympathetic tone and promoting relaxation. This leads to reduced heart rate, improved sleep quality, and lowered cortisol levels. Improved autonomic regulation is essential in older adults, many of whom suffer from insomnia, hypertension, or anxiety. Warming the body mildly increases metabolic rate, which can enhance tissue oxygenation and enzyme activity during rehabilitation. This promotes better cellular repair in aged tissues with slower healing dynamics.

5.1.2 Contrast therapy and cold water applications (10–20°C)

In some cases, cold or alternating hot-cold therapy (contrast hydrotherapy) is used for older adults with acute inflammation, swelling, or vascular dysfunction:

- Cold water (10–20°C) induces vasoconstriction, helping reduce inflammation, joint effusion, and delayed-onset muscle soreness after physical activity.
- Contrast hydrotherapy (alternating immersion in hot and cold water) triggers a vascular pumping effect, which can enhance lymphatic drainage and circulation, useful in managing venous insufficiency or chronic oedema.

However, cold therapy should be used cautiously in older individuals due to their reduced thermoregulatory capacity and potential for cold intolerance or cardiovascular instability [48].

5.1.3 Therapeutic customisation based on comorbidity

The choice of hydrotherapy temperature should always be individualised in geriatric patients [49]. For example:

- Warmer temperatures (35–36°C) are ideal for those with osteoarthritis, chronic back pain, or fibromyalgia to promote muscle relaxation and pain relief.
- Moderate temperatures (31–33°C) are used for cardiopulmonary compromised elderly, ensuring safe haemodynamic response during aerobic aquatic activity.
- Cooler ranges (27–29°C) may be utilised in higher-intensity aquatic exercise where heat stress or fatigue must be minimised.

The thermodynamic properties of water—particularly warm water—are central to hydrotherapy's clinical utility in geriatric rehabilitation. By harnessing these thermal effects, clinicians can address pain, stiffness, circulation, and neuromuscular tone holistically. Warm water immersion offers a low-risk, high-benefit intervention for ageing populations who often face limitations in conventional physiotherapy. When designed with accessibility, individualised protocols, and safety in mind, hydrotherapy becomes a cornerstone modality for promoting functional independence and quality of life in older adults [3, 47, 50].

5.2 The therapeutic triad in aquatic therapy

Aquatic therapy utilises the unique mechanical properties of water—buoyancy, viscosity, and hydrostatic pressure—to create a safe, effective, and therapeutic environment, especially beneficial for elderly individuals or those with physical impairments.

5.2.1 Buoyancy: Reducing load, enabling movement

Buoyancy is governed by Archimedes' principle, which states that any object submerged in a fluid is acted upon by an upward force equal to the weight of the fluid displaced. In practical terms, this means that the body experiences a reduction in gravitational load when immersed in water. According to Becker [3], immersion to the level of the xiphoid process (mid-chest) reduces effective body weight by approximately 60%, while immersion to the neck can reduce it by nearly 90% [3].

This offloading effect significantly decreases joint compression forces, making it easier for individuals with arthritis, osteoporosis, or general frailty to perform movements that would otherwise be painful or impossible on land. It encourages mobility, improves joint range of motion, and reduces pain without the risk of fall-related injuries. Thus, buoyancy allows for safe and supportive rehabilitation, particularly for the elderly or those recovering from musculoskeletal injuries.

5.2.2 Viscosity: Natural resistance for strength and control

Viscosity refers to the internal friction within the water that resists the movement of objects through it. Unlike static weights or fixed resistance machines on land, water provides constant, multidirectional, and self-adjusting resistance. The faster or larger the movement, the greater the resistance encountered. This unique property allows individuals to tailor the intensity of exercise subconsciously based on their capabilities.

A research article highlighted that this natural resistance helps improve muscle strength, coordination, and balance, all within a safe, low-impact environment. Importantly, it also promotes motor learning and neuromuscular control, which are essential for elderly individuals with impaired proprioception, sarcopenia, or balance disorders [51]. Furthermore, resistance training in water helps to preserve lean muscle mass and functionality, which is crucial for improving balance responses during unexpected movements or falls, ultimately supporting independence in older adults [52].

5.2.3 Hydrostatic pressure: Enhancing circulation and stability

Hydrostatic pressure is the uniform force exerted by water on the body's surface, increasing with depth. This pressure acts as a gentle compression garment, aiding in venous return, reducing limb oedema, and stabilising joints during movement. It provides a key circulatory benefit for elderly individuals suffering from chronic venous insufficiency, varicose veins, or orthostatic intolerance.

The hydrostatic pressure supports haemodynamic stability, improves cardiovascular efficiency, and reduces the orthostatic load, making it easier for individuals to exercise without dizziness or fatigue [53]. Additionally, the pressure stimulates cutaneous and proprioceptive receptors, enhancing sensory feedback. This is particularly beneficial for individuals with diabetic neuropathy, vestibular dysfunction, or impaired motor control, as their reduced sensory integration makes improvements in balance, walking efficiency, and overall independence especially impactful [54].

6. Therapeutic water-based interventions for the elderly

As ageing populations grow worldwide, so does the need for safe, effective, and adaptable rehabilitation methods. Hydrotherapy—the use of water for therapeutic purposes—has emerged as a powerful intervention for older adults, especially those facing chronic pain, reduced mobility, cardiovascular limitations, or musculoskeletal degeneration. Various types of hydrotherapy offer targeted physiological and psychological benefits by leveraging water's inherent mechanical and thermal properties such as buoyancy, viscosity, hydrostatic pressure, and thermal conductivity [3]. This chapter outlines five evidence-supported hydrotherapy modalities that are particularly suitable for elderly individuals.

6.1 Warm water pool therapy

Warm water pool therapy, also referred to as aquatic physical therapy or balneotherapy, involves performing therapeutic exercises in a temperature-controlled pool, typically maintained between 32°C and 34°C (89.6–93.2°F). This modality utilises buoyancy to reduce joint loading, viscosity for gentle resistance, and warmth to relax muscles and increase blood flow [7]. For older adults with osteoarthritis, rheumatoid arthritis, osteoporosis, or generalised frailty, warm water immersion significantly reduces pain and stiffness, enhancing joint mobility and functional independence [55]. The thermal effect also stimulates parasympathetic activity, aiding in stress relief and improved sleep quality. According to Becker [3], immersion to chest depth reduces weight bearing by up to 60%, allowing elderly individuals to perform movement without the fear of falling or pain-induced hesitation. Additionally, warm water therapy enhances cardiovascular function without the overexertion commonly associated with land-based aerobic exercises, making it a safe choice for individuals with mild to moderate cardiac conditions.

6.2 Aquatic Tai Chi or Ai Chi

Aquatic Tai Chi and water-based yoga combine the benefits of slow, mindful movement with the therapeutic environment of warm water. These practices emphasise balance, breath control, flexibility, and mental focus, making them ideal for elderly individuals with postural instability, cognitive decline, or chronic stress. The buoyancy of water supports slow, fluid movements, allowing older adults with joint limitations, Parkinson's disease, or post-stroke conditions to participate without overexertion. According to Tsang and Hui-Chan [56], aquatic Tai Chi significantly improved balance control and reduced the risk of falls in older individuals. Moreover, the meditative aspect of aquatic yoga or Tai Chi enhances mind-body awareness, promoting parasympathetic dominance, reducing anxiety, and improving mood [57]. Such interventions are especially valuable in combating social isolation and depression, common challenges in ageing populations.

6.3 Deep water walking/treadmill and resistance therapy

Technological advancements in hydrotherapy have introduced the use of underwater treadmills and adjustable resistance jets, allowing precise control of exercise intensity in a safe, supportive medium. Walking or jogging on a submerged treadmill reduces the impact on joints while still providing cardiovascular and musculoskeletal benefits (**Figure 3**) [58]. This form of therapy is highly suitable for elderly patients recovering from hip or knee replacements or those with sarcopenia and gait abnormalities. The water's resistance challenges multiple muscle groups while simultaneously enhancing proprioception and balance control. Resistance jets can be adjusted

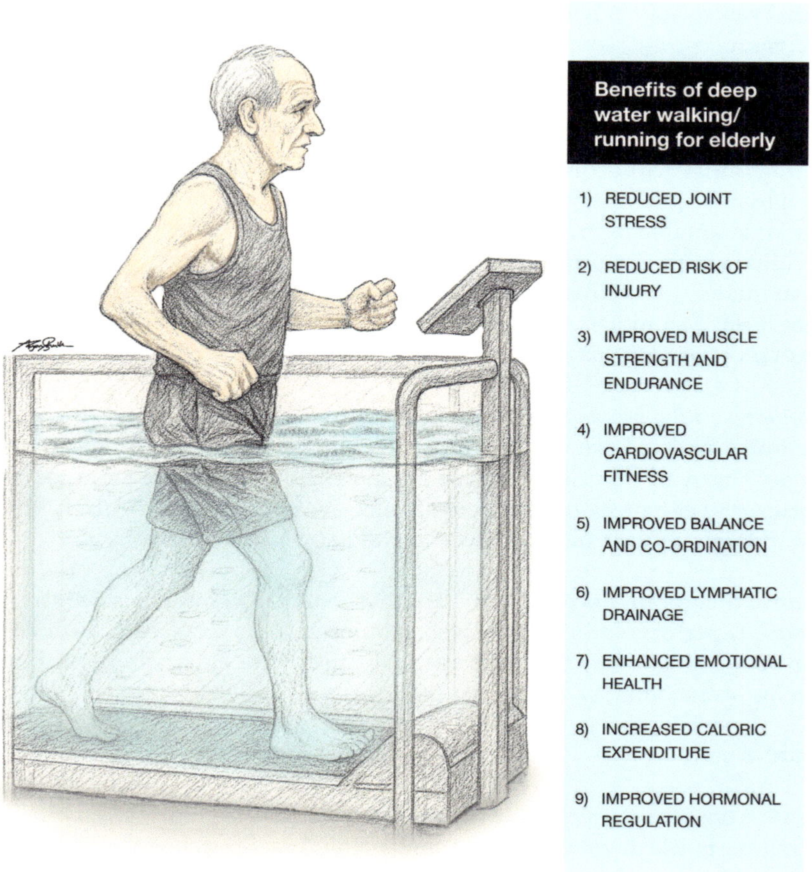

Figure 3.
The benefits of deep-water walking on an aqua treadmill for the elderly [58, 59].

to create tailored strength-building regimens, encouraging neuromuscular coordination and endurance [59]. In studies involving geriatric patients with chronic mobility impairments, regular underwater treadmill sessions were shown to improve stride length, walking speed, and muscle activation patterns, which are vital indicators for fall risk reduction [60].

6.4 Immersion therapy for lymphatic and venous return

Static immersion therapy, where an individual remains passively submerged in warm water up to neck or chest level, leverages hydrostatic pressure to promote venous return, reduce oedema, and support lymphatic flow. This is especially beneficial for elderly patients with congestive heart failure, lymphedema, or chronic leg swelling [61]. Hydrostatic pressure, which increases with depth, compresses the limbs uniformly and enhances the movement of extracellular fluids, effectively reducing swelling and aiding circulation. This results in decreased discomfort, improved lower limb mobility, and prevention of venous pooling, a common issue in sedentary or immobile seniors [62]. Additionally, static immersion contributes to deep relaxation, lowering blood pressure and heart rate, while supporting cognitive clarity and emotional well-being. When used regularly, it becomes a valuable tool in the management of vascular conditions and stress-related physiological strain.

6.5 Hydrogymnastics

Hydrogymnastics encompasses a range of water-based therapeutic exercises designed to improve cardiovascular fitness, strength, balance, and mobility. This modality is adaptable to various age groups, including the elderly, and can be tailored to individual needs. A study by Lima et al. [63] found that hydrogymnastics promoted an increase in agility and leg muscle strength in elderly women despite the low evidence level. Techniques such as the Bad Ragaz Ring Method (BRRM) and Watsu are integral components of hydrogymnastics.

- *Bad Ragaz Ring Method (BRRM):* Originating from Switzerland, BRRM involves therapist-assisted exercises performed while the patient is supported by flotation rings. This method utilises proprioceptive neuromuscular facilitation (PNF) patterns to enhance neuromuscular function, making it particularly beneficial for individuals with musculoskeletal and neurological conditions.

- *Watsu:* A combination of water-based Shiatsu massage and passive stretching. Watsu is performed in warm water, promoting deep relaxation, pain relief, and improved range of motion. It is especially useful for elderly individuals experiencing stress, anxiety, or chronic pain.

6.6 AquaStretch

AquaStretch is a relatively new technique that involves guided stretching and myofascial release in warm water. A study comparing AquaStretch with supervised land-based stretching found that AquaStretch was beneficial in reducing pain and disability [64]. The process includes four steps: play (exploring movements), freeze (identifying areas of restriction), pressure (applying manual pressure), and move (performing movements to release tension). This method has shown promise in reducing pain and improving flexibility among older adults with musculoskeletal issues.

6.7 Hydromassage

Hydromassage utilises water jets to deliver targeted massage therapy, promoting relaxation, pain relief, and improved circulation. This non-invasive technique is particularly beneficial for seniors, as it alleviates muscle tension and enhances mobility without placing additional strain on the body. The warmth of the water further contributes to muscle relaxation and stress reduction. HydroWorx highlights that hydromassage can enhance mobility and flexibility in ageing adults, contributing to overall wellness [65].

The evolution of hydrotherapy has introduced a variety of innovative techniques that cater to the unique needs of the ageing population. From traditional methods like hydrogymnastics and immersion therapy to cutting-edge technologies such as VR integration and smart monitoring devices, these modalities offer comprehensive benefits that address both physical and psychological aspects of health [66, 67]. Incorporating these therapies into geriatric care can significantly enhance mobility, reduce pain, and improve the overall quality of life for older adults.

7. Hydrotherapy: A scientific pillar in the prevention and regeneration of age-associated decline

The global ageing population is experiencing an increase in chronic, degenerative, and lifestyle-related diseases. Conditions such as cardiovascular disease, type 2 diabetes, osteoporosis, arthritis, neurodegenerative disorders, and respiratory illnesses are common among the elderly and contribute to reduced quality of life and increased healthcare burden. Preventing the onset or progression of these diseases through result-driven interventions is a vital public health priority. Ageing is associated with physiological changes that increase vulnerability to multiple diseases. These include reduced muscle mass, diminished immune function, hormonal imbalances, decreased mobility, and impaired metabolic function. When combined with sedentary lifestyles, poor nutrition, environmental stressors, and social isolation, these factors significantly elevate disease risk.

7.1 Global standard preventive strategies for senior citizens: Health education and literacy programmes

Educate older adults about ageing-related health risks and prevention strategies. Use age-appropriate communication in local languages, visual aids, and interactive sessions. Promote self-care practices, medication management, and health-seeking behaviour [68].

7.2 Routine health screening and early detection

Community-based screening for hypertension, diabetes, osteoporosis, vision, hearing, and cognitive decline. Integration of mobile clinics and primary health workers for home visits.

7.3 Physical activity and mobility programmes

Promote structured, supervised physical activity programmes such as walking clubs, Tai Chi, and chair exercises. Include fall prevention training and balance exercises to reduce injury risk.

7.4 Nutritional support and counselling

Facilitate community kitchens and meal delivery with nutrient-dense options. Provide individual or group dietary counselling focused on age-appropriate nutrition [69].

7.5 Social engagement and mental health promotion

Foster social participation through community centres, hobby groups, and volunteering opportunities. Train peer counsellors and social workers to detect and support cases of depression, anxiety, or dementia [70].

7.6 Environmental and safety intervention

Modify public and home environments to reduce fall risk (e.g., handrails, ramps, and non-slip flooring). Ensure accessible transportation and safe community spaces for the elderly.

7.7 Concept of bridging the global divide of the prevention and regeneration in elderly care

As the global population continues to age, the demand for preventive and regenerative healthcare interventions is reaching a critical point. Yet, a significant implementation gap exists globally—especially in low- and middle-income countries—between what is scientifically possible and what is systemically delivered. Despite evidence-based interventions available for delaying age-associated decline, their integration into mainstream care is far from optimal. Hydrotherapy, the therapeutic use of water, has long been recognised for its benefits in rehabilitation and wellness. For the elderly, it offers a gentle yet effective means to address various physical and mental health challenges. To maximise its potential, a strategic approach involving medical education, clinical integration, community awareness, and collaborative efforts is essential.

7.8 The prevention gap

Preventive care for older adults remains alarmingly under-addressed on the global stage. According to the World Health Organisation, out of 194 member countries, only 63% have strategies specifically focused on ageing, and merely 54% have national action plans for older adults' health [71]. Even fewer have policies to address ageism or establish long-term care systems, which directly affects the quality of life in ageing population [72]. This lack of infrastructure and policy results in a rise in avoidable chronic conditions, including sarcopenia, falls, cardiovascular strain, and neurocognitive decline. Preventive care models—such as routine movement assessments, nutritional support, and fall prevention strategies—are either inconsistently implemented or absent, particularly in resource-limited settings.

7.9 The regeneration shortfall

While regenerative medicine, rehabilitation, and therapies like hydrotherapy, neuroplasticity-focused interventions, and resistance-based rehab are advancing, access remains uneven. Most older adults in underprivileged family backgrounds have limited access to even basic rehabilitation services, let alone advanced regenerative protocols. According to the World Bank, healthcare systems across developing countries are "not designed for the complex, long-term needs of aging adults," often citing cost, medication access, and transportation as key barriers [73].

7.10 The policy mandate: WHO's decade of healthy ageing

The WHO Decade of Healthy Ageing (2021–2030) [74] presents a comprehensive framework for action, urging nations to invest in four priority areas:

1. Changing perceptions of ageing,

2. Integrated care for older adults,

3. Age-friendly environments, and

4. Improved access to long-term care.

Yet, execution remains a bottleneck. Without cross-sectoral collaboration, adequate funding, and primary care reform, this ambitious framework may fall short of its goals [75].

Hydrotherapy, the therapeutic use of water for physical and psychological healing, is an underutilised yet powerful modality in modern medicine. As the global population ages and chronic lifestyle diseases become increasingly prevalent, the need for non-invasive, cost-effective, and holistic interventions like hydrotherapy is growing. Integrating hydrotherapy into clinical prescriptions and expanding its educational, infrastructural, and social presence can serve as a pivotal step in bridging the gap between prevention and regeneration in healthcare. The first essential step is the inclusion of hydrotherapy in medical education. By incorporating the science and techniques of hydrotherapy into undergraduate medical and physiotherapy curriculum, we can empower future healthcare professionals with the knowledge to prescribe and utilise it effectively. This foundational knowledge not only enhances clinical decision-making but also improves the generalisability and consistency of hydrotherapy practices across diverse healthcare settings. When doctors, physiotherapists, and rehabilitation specialists are uniformly trained in hydrotherapy protocols, it reduces variability in care and boosts patient confidence in these non-pharmacological interventions. Beyond the clinical setting, raising public awareness especially among the elderly is equally critical. Many senior citizens suffer from joint pain, reduced mobility, anxiety and metabolic conditions, all of which can be positively influenced by water-based therapies. However, a significant portion of this population remains unaware of hydrotherapy's benefits. Educational campaigns, workshops,

Sr. no.	Domain	Strategy	Impact
(1)	Medical education and research	Introduce hydrotherapy in MBBS and physiotherapy curricula	Builds foundational knowledge and clinical confidence among future healthcare providers
(2)	Clinical prescription	Integrate hydrotherapy protocols into routine prescriptions for elderly and rehabilitation patients	Enhances outcomes in pain management, mobility, and mental health
(3)	Community awareness	Run campaigns and workshops for the elderly about hydrotherapy benefits	Improves utilisation and self-care participation among ageing populations
(4)	NGO and fundraiser	Partner with NGOs and health funders to create affordable hydrotherapy access in low-resource areas	Reduces health inequality; reaches underprivileged elderly populations
(5)	Local facility promotion	Establish small-scale local hydrotherapy units and hold educational camps	Provides practical access and knowledge reinforcement within communities
(6)	Policy level advocacy	Advocate for hydrotherapy inclusion in public healthcare protocols and insurance coverage	Institutionalises hydrotherapy in mainstream healthcare infrastructure
(7)	International collaboration	Share data and practices with global institutions to standardise hydrotherapy across nations	Contributes to a global preventive and regenerative care model

Table 3.
Strategic framework for integrating hydrotherapy in clinical and community health system [76].

and community programmes can help older adults understand how hydrotherapy supports both mental and physical well-being, leading to improved quality of life and reduced healthcare dependency. Equity in healthcare access is another important pillar. Collaborating with NGOs, charitable trusts, and healthcare fundraisers can help bring hydrotherapy to the doorsteps of the underprivileged, particularly through government health infrastructure. This approach ensures that the benefits of this therapy are not confined to urban elite hospitals but are made available to rural and low-income populations who may lack access to advanced medical treatments. For example, mobile hydrotherapy units or partnerships with public health centres could serve as practical and scalable solutions.

Additionally, promoting hydrotherapy through local facilities, digital media, and knowledge camps can further improve community engagement. When people see real-life stories, testimonials, and local success models, they are more likely to try such therapies themselves. Interactive media campaigns and village or town-level hydrotherapy awareness camps can raise the knowledge baseline within a community, sparking long-term shifts in health-seeking behaviours. Finally, scaling this movement nationally and internationally will amplify its impact. Through policy support, international collaboration, and inclusion in public health initiatives, hydrotherapy can evolve from an ancillary therapy to a mainstream pillar of preventive and regenerative healthcare. When these strategies converge education, awareness, accessibility, and policy, hydrotherapy can offer not just relief but resilience, especially for the ageing global population. In summary, hydrotherapy is not merely a treatment, and it is a potential foundation for a healthcare model rooted in prevention, accessibility, and regeneration. With structured integration, we can create a system where healing begins before disease even takes hold (**Table 3**) [76].

8. Comparative efficacy: Hydrotherapy versus land-based exercise in geriatrics

As the global demographic continues to shift towards an older population, preserving functional independence and reducing fall risk have become critical priorities in geriatric healthcare. Both hydrotherapy (water-based therapeutic exercise) and traditional land-based exercise are commonly employed to improve balance, mobility, and overall well-being in older adults. This section explores current research comparing the effectiveness of these two approaches, with particular emphasis on functional performance, balance enhancement, fall prevention, and patient adherence and satisfaction levels. Additionally, it highlights the necessity of individualised, strategic intervention planning, acknowledging that no single method is universally superior for all patients.

8.1 Functional outcomes and balance improvement

Recent studies have explored the comparative effects of hydrotherapy and land-based exercise on functional outcomes in older adults (**Table 4**). A systematic review and meta-analysis by Zhang et al. [80] included 29 randomised controlled trials (RCTs) with 1486 older adults. The analysis revealed that aquatic-based exercise (AE) significantly improved balance ability, as measured by the Berg Balance Scale (BBS) and the 30-second chair stand test.

However, no significant differences were found between AE and LE in terms of the 6-minute walking test and the Timed Up and Go Test (TUGT), suggesting that both

Sr. no	Parameter	Land-based physiotherapy	Water-based physiotherapy
(1)	Balance and fall risk	Higher fall risk during exercise sessions	Lower fall risk due to water support and multidirectional resistance
(2)	Joint load and impact	Higher mechanical load; may aggravate joint pain or arthritis in some individuals	Reduced load due to buoyancy; safer for individuals with joint pain or reduced mobility
(3)	Muscle strength	Effective for weight-bearing and resistance training	Effective due to water resistance; gentler yet comprehensive strengthening
(4)	Cardiovascular demand	Moderate to high depending on intensity; may need careful monitoring	Water immersion enhances stroke volume with lower heart rate during activity
(5)	Neurological function	Enhances proprioception but may cause anxiety in frail patients	Water environment stimulates sensory feedback and promotes psychological comfort
(6)	Thermal effects	No thermal benefit unless used with adjunctive modalities (infrared heat panels)	Warm water improves circulation, reduces spasticity, and supports muscle relaxation
(7)	Accessibility and infrastructure	Easily available in most physiotherapy clinics	Requires access to therapeutic pools and specialised staff
(8)	Exercise adherence and participation	May be lower due to fear of falling or joint discomfort	Often higher due to pain reduction, sense of confidence and enjoyment in aquatic environments

Table 4.
Comparative analysis of land-based and water-based physiotherapy in older adults, highlighting therapeutic and psychosocial benefits supported by systematic review and meta-analysis evidence [77–79].

modalities are effective in enhancing certain aspects of balance and mobility. In a randomised controlled trial focusing on community-dwelling elderly individuals with a history of falling, both water-based and land-based exercise groups showed significant improvements in hip abduction and adduction strength. Quality of life (QOL) measures also improved in both groups, with no significant differences between them, indicating that both exercise modalities are beneficial for physical function and psychological well-being [81].

8.2 Fall prevention

Fall prevention is a critical concern in geriatric health. A systematic review by Thomas et al. [82] examined various physical activity programmes for balance and fall prevention in the elderly. The review concluded that both aquatic and land-based exercises effectively reduce fall risk, with no clear superiority of one over the other. The choice between modalities should be based on individual preferences, physical abilities, and access to facilities.

8.3 Patient adherence and satisfaction

Adherence to exercise programmes is essential for achieving desired health outcomes. A systematic review and meta-analysis by Osho et al. [83] found that group-based fall prevention exercise programmes had an average adherence rate of around

66%, with lower adherence observed in programmes that were highly repetitive or of long duration. The supportive and enjoyable environment of aquatic exercises may enhance adherence, especially among individuals who find land-based exercises challenging or monotonous.

8.4 Strategic planning of interventions

The effectiveness of exercise interventions in geriatric populations depends on strategic planning tailored to individual needs. Factors such as medical history, physical capabilities, psychological readiness, and environmental considerations should guide the selection of exercise modalities. By adopting a versatile and flexible approach, healthcare providers can effectively utilise both hydrotherapy and land-based exercises to promote active ageing and reduce the risk of falls in the geriatric population. For instance, individuals with joint pain or mobility limitations may benefit more from the low-impact nature of hydrotherapy, while those aiming to improve weight-bearing strength might prefer land-based exercises. Moreover, integrating both hydrotherapy and land-based exercises in a complementary manner could address a broader range of functional goals. For example, starting with hydrotherapy to build confidence and reduce pain, followed by land-based exercises to enhance strength and endurance, may offer a balanced approach to rehabilitation.

8.4.1 Changing the trend of degeneration and deconditioning through water-based practices

Ageing is accompanied by progressive biological shifts leading to physical decline, diminished cardiovascular function, and neuroplastic changes. These biological shifts are often accelerated by a sedentary lifestyle, resulting in what is termed "physical deconditioning," a reversible decline in physical performance due to inactivity [84]. Water-based therapy has shown promise in reversing or slowing these degenerative changes. In a systematic review by Barker et al. [85, 86], aquatic exercises were associated with significant improvements in lower limb strength, endurance, and balance in older adults. The resistance provided by water allows for muscle activation comparable to land-based exercise without the mechanical load on joints. Further, aquatic training can help preserve bone mineral density, improve gait mechanics, and reduce the risk of sarcopenia [87]. These outcomes are crucial in delaying institutionalisation and enhancing the quality of independent life in ageing populations.

8.4.2 Promoting neuroplasticity and active ageing

Engaging in novel and multi-sensory environments such as water stimulates the brain, supporting cognitive-motor integration and neuroplasticity. Regular aquatic exercise has been shown to improve executive function, spatial awareness, and dual-task processing in the elderly [88]. Water-based therapy requires constant postural control and sensory recalibration, stimulating the vestibular and proprioceptive systems more dynamically than land-based routines. This concept aligns with the "Use it or lose it" principle in active ageing, suggesting that consistent engagement in complex, enjoyable tasks like hydrotherapy can slow neurocognitive decline and promote emotional well-being [89]. Aquatic exercise has systemic anti-inflammatory effects. Chronic inflammation plays a major role in age-related diseases such as cardiovascular disease, diabetes, and neurodegeneration. A study by Nagle et al. [90] found that moderate aquatic exercise significantly reduced C-reactive protein (CRP) levels and interleukin-6, two markers linked to systemic inflammation. Additionally, aquatic therapy improves insulin sensitivity, lipid profiles, and blood pressure, contributing to metabolic health in elderly individuals with conditions like type 2 diabetes or metabolic syndrome [91]. The thermoregulatory environment of warm water further enhances circulation and parasympathetic tone, supporting autonomic balance and hormonal regulation.

8.4.3 Integrating hydrotherapy into geriatric routines

A well-defined framework is necessary to ensure that hydrotherapy transitions from an occasional therapeutic tool to a sustainable and culturally integrated practice in geriatric care. Creating low-barrier access to hydrotherapy through regular sessions embedded into weekly schedules helps build habit formation. A proposed routine should include two to three aquatic sessions per week, each 30–45 minutes, with an alternating focus on strength, balance, and relaxation, with Post-exercise recovery periods emphasising stretching and breathing. For institutionalised or home-based elderly individuals, portable pools or shared community spaces can serve as intervention points. Hydrotherapy can be adapted for group formats or individualised home-based programmes by educating geriatric caregivers and family members. Sustaining hydrotherapy benefits requires the education of caregivers and family units, especially in cultures where ageing is managed at home. Education sessions for caregivers and family members should include signs of mental and physical fatigue in the elderly, learning safe aquatic movements and understanding contraindications and emergency protocols. Digital toolkits, videos, and on-site workshops can equip caregivers with knowledge and confidence. As caregivers become facilitators, they help reinforce behavioural continuity, increasing programme retention and efficacy [92].

8.4.4 Sustainable long-term adherence strategies

To maintain participation, programmes must prioritise enjoyment, relevance, and social engagement. This includes Incorporating music, games, and social challenges, Providing progress tracking to celebrate small wins and offering incentives or community recognition. Sustainability also depends on policy support. Governments, NGOs, and health organisations should prioritise funding for hydrotherapy infrastructure and incorporate it into public health models. Additionally, tele-hydrotherapy—with virtual coaching and AI monitoring—can expand access to remote or mobility-challenged populations. Group-based hydrotherapy sessions also promote social inclusion. Elderly individuals, especially those living alone or with limited mobility, often face isolation. Structured group hydrotherapy facilitates community engagement, social interaction, and psychological upliftment. A study by Vivas et al. [93] found that social bonding in aquatic classes enhanced adherence and psychological well-being, contributing to reduced depressive symptoms. Furthermore, social inclusion supports active and dignified ageing. Empowering elderly individuals to take charge of their own rehabilitation fosters a sense of autonomy. The buoyancy of water enables pain-free movement, even in those with severe arthritis or neuromuscular conditions, offering a sense of possibility often absent in land-based therapy.

8.4.5 Scope for research, innovation, and policy integration

Future advancements in hydrotherapy depend on robust research, technological innovation, and progressive health policies. Smart aquatic technologies, such as underwater gait analysis, wearable hydro-stable heart rate monitors, and temperature-controlled resistance systems, are emerging as tools to enhance precision and safety in aquatic therapy. These innovations allow for personalised programming and progress monitoring, which is essential for high-risk elderly populations [94]. Virtual hydrotherapy through AR/VR is another frontier, especially for individuals without access to aquatic centres. Immersive environments can simulate the soothing and exercise effects of water through neurofeedback and bio-mimetic interfaces. From a policy standpoint, there is an urgent need for guidelines and funding mechanisms that prioritise ageing-inclusive wellness infrastructure. Public-private partnerships, NGO involvement, and urban planning that incorporates hydrotherapy pools in senior living communities are promising steps. Governments can support this by integrating hydrotherapy within health insurance reimbursement models, thereby increasing uptake across socioeconomic strata. Research-wise, there remains a deficit of high-quality randomised controlled trials (RCTs) that compare hydrotherapy with other interventions across various ageing-related conditions (e.g., frailty, cognitive decline, and post-surgical rehab). Systematic reviews, such as that by Waller et al. [95], call for standardisation in outcome measures, dosage, and follow-up duration to enhance meta-analytic validity.

9. The next frontier in elder care and active ageing

True societal advancement is measured not by how long people live but by how well they live, maintaining autonomy, functional capacity, and emotional well-being. To conclude, this chapter has traced the growing concerns in geriatric health, unravelling the biological and psychosocial contributors to the decline while offering strategic solutions aimed at restoring vitality. Central to this evolving framework is an often overlooked yet highly effective therapeutic option: hydrotherapy. Hydrotherapy uniquely combines multiple physiological and psychological benefits supporting muscle strength, cardiovascular health, sensory integration, and emotional resilience, all within a low-impact, buoyant, and interactive aquatic setting. For older adults affected by conditions such as sarcopenia, frailty, fall risk, chronic pain, or social disconnection, hydrotherapy is more than an adjunct. It is a regenerative and preventive intervention that aligns with the complex needs of ageing individuals. Its evidence-based effects on mobility, balance, and psychological well-being make it a cornerstone of comprehensive geriatric care.

With intentional, well-structured implementation, hydrotherapy can be seamlessly incorporated into daily or weekly regimens, customised for vulnerable or high-risk groups, and scaled from specialised clinics to community centres and home-based models. It allows elderly individuals to engage in physical activity without fear, fosters social participation, and rebuilds a sense of bodily trust and mental assurance. The water's ability to reduce systemic inflammation, support neuro-dynamic changes, and counteract degenerative processes marks a fundamental shift from reactive healthcare to preventive and restorative ageing solutions [96]. In conclusion, hydrotherapy is not merely a tool; it is a philosophy. A gentle, immersive path that honours the ageing body, respects its limitations, and unlocks its potential. Let this chapter not only inform but inspire a paradigm shift: from rigid land-based assumptions to fluid, inclusive, and empowering water-based care. With hydrotherapy, we do not just extend life; we enrich it, reclaim it, and celebrate it. The time to act is now. The future of ageing begins in water.

Acknowledgements

I extend my deepest gratitude to the elderly patients who graciously shared their journeys and inspired the essence of this chapter. Their resilience and trust have been the cornerstone of my research and writing. I am sincerely thankful to my mentors and fellow specialists whose guidance and wisdom helped shape the scientific foundation of this work. Their support at critical junctures strengthened my resolve and refined my understanding. To my father, Sanjeev M. Shukla, your unwavering belief in my purpose and your powerful reminder that my research and words have the potential to plant seeds of transformation in society has been my greatest motivation whenever I faced barriers. You have taught me the value of perseverance with purpose. I also wish to thank myself—for staying disciplined, dedicated, and committed to reading, learning, and working for the welfare of my patients. This journey has been as much internal as it is academic. I will continue to write with the hope of educating students and serving the global community. May this chapter find its way into the hands of those who seek meaning, knowledge, and change. The author acknowledges the use of Artificial intelligence through ChatGPT 4.1 for the polishing of the language.

Author details

Aryan Shukla
Senior Sports, Physiotherapist, Mumbai, India

*Address all correspondence to: dr.muscle960@icloud.com

References

[1] World Health Organization (WHO). Decade of Healthy Ageing: Baseline Report. Geneva: WHO; 2021

[2] Cruz-Jentoft AJ et al. Sarcopenia: Revised European consensus on definition and diagnosis. Age and Ageing. 2019;**48**(1):16-31

[3] Becker BE. Aquatic therapy: Scientific foundations and clinical rehabilitation applications. PM & R: The Journal of Injury, Function, and Rehabilitation. 2009;**1**(9):859-872

[4] Kamioka H et al. Effectiveness of aquatic exercise and balneotherapy: A summary of systematic reviews based on randomized controlled trials of water immersion therapies. Journal of Epidemiology. 2010;**20**(1):2-12

[5] Vivas J, Arias P, Cudeiro J. Aquatic therapy in elderly balance rehabilitation: A meta-analysis. Aging Clinical and Experimental Research. 2023;**35**(4):645-655

[6] Noh DK, Lim JY, Shin HI, Paik NJ. The effect of aquatic therapy on postural balance and muscle strength in stroke survivors. Journal of Physical Therapy Science. 2008;**20**(1):43-48

[7] Geytenbeek JJ. Evidence for effective hydrotherapy. Physiotherapy. 2002;**88**(9):514-529

[8] Mathers CD, Stevens GA, Boerma T, et al. Global and regional causes of death: Patterns and trends, 2000-2015. The Lancet Global Health. 2015;**3**(10):e593-e603

[9] Watson KB, Wiltz JL, Nhim K, Kaufmann RB, Thomas CW, Greenlund KJ. Trends in multiple chronic conditions among US adults, by life stage, behavioral risk factor surveillance system, 2013-2023. Preventing Chronic Disease. 2025;**22**:E15. DOI: 10.5888/pcd22.240539

[10] Inouye SK, Studenski S, Tinetti ME, Kuchel GA. Geriatric syndromes: Clinical, research, and policy implications of a core geriatric concept. Journal of the American Geriatrics Society. 2007;**55**(5):780-791

[11] Fried LP, Tangen CM, et al. Frailty in older adults: Evidence for a phenotype. Journal of Gerontology: Medical Sciences. 2001;**56**(3):M146-M157

[12] Ambrose AF, Paul G, Hausdorff JM. Risk factors for falls among older adults: A review of the literature. Maturitas. 2013;**75**(1):51-61

[13] Fries JF. Aging, natural death, and the compression of morbidity. New England Journal of Medicine. 1980;**303**(3):130-135

[14] Holt-Lunstad J, Smith TB, Layton JB. Social relationships and mortality risk: A meta-analytic review. PLoS Medicine. 2010;**7**(7):e1000316

[15] WHO. World Report on Ageing and Health. 2020. Available from: https://www.who.int/ageing/publications/world-report-2015/en/

[16] United Nations, Department of Economic and Social Affairs, Population Division. World Population Prospects 2022: Summary of Results. United Nations; 2022. 52 pages. ISBN: 978-92-1-001438-0. DOI: 10.18356/9789210014380

[17] Centers for Disease Control and Prevention. Demographic Differences

in Life Dissatisfaction Among Adults: United States, 2021. National Health Statistics Reports, Number 192. Hyattsville, MD: National Center for Health Statistics; 2023. 12 p. Available from: NCHS digital release

[18] Ziaaldini MM, Fathi R, Dabidi Roshan V. Sarcopenia and its molecular mechanisms in aging and physical inactivity: A narrative review. Frontiers in Physiology. 2022;**13**:972511. DOI: 10.3389/fphys.2022.972511

[19] Di Girolamo FG, Situlin R, Mazzucco S, Valentini R, Toigo G, Biolo G. Protein metabolism and exercise in the elderly: A narrative review. Aging Clinical and Experimental Research. 2021;**33**(4):895-903. DOI: 10.1007/s40520-021-01803-x

[20] Joseph AM, Adhihetty PJ, Buford TW, Wohlgemuth SE, Lees HA, Nguyen LM, et al. The impact of aging on mitochondrial function and biogenesis pathways in skeletal muscle of sedentary high- and low-functioning elderly individuals. Aging Cell. 2013;**12**(5):851-862. DOI: 10.1111/acel.12102

[21] Loeser RF. Aging and osteoarthritis: The role of chondrocyte senescence and aging changes in the cartilage matrix. Osteoarthritis and Cartilage. 2009;**17**(8):971-979. DOI: 10.1016/j.joca.2009.03.002

[22] Kuiper JS, Zuidersma M, Oude Voshaar RC, Zuidema SU, van den Heuvel ER, Stolk RP, et al. Social relationships and risk of dementia: A systematic review and meta-analysis of longitudinal cohort studies. Ageing Research Reviews. 2016;**22**:39-57. DOI: 10.1016/j.arr.2015.04.006

[23] Shen Y, Li S, Li W, Wang C, Meng X. Global prevalence and risk factors of depression and anxiety among older adults: A systematic review and meta-analysis. BMC Geriatrics. 2024;**24**:71

[24] Flaatten H, Beil M, Guidet B, The VIP2 Study Group. The challenge of the older ICU patient. International Journal of Critical Illness and Injury Science. 2021;**11**(2):64-71. DOI: 10.4103/IJCIIS.IJCIIS_104_20

[25] Adelman RD, Tmanova LL, Delgado D, Dion S, Lachs MS. Caregiver burden: A clinical review. JAMA. 2014;**311**(10):1052-1060. DOI: 10.1001/jama.2014.304

[26] Maher RL, Hanlon J, Hajjar ER. Clinical consequences of polypharmacy in elderly. Expert Opinion on Drug Safety. 2014;**13**(1):57-65

[27] Zia A, Kamaruzzaman SB, Tan MP. Polypharmacy and falls in older people: Balancing evidence-based medicine against falls risk. Postgraduate Medicine. 2020;**132**(3):248-257

[28] Hilmer SN, Gnjidic D. The effects of polypharmacy in older adults. Clinical Pharmacology and Therapeutics. 2009;**85**(1):86-88

[29] Engel GL. The need for a new medical model: A challenge for biomedicine. Science. 1977;**196**(4286):129-136

[30] Lawton MP. The Philadelphia geriatric center morale scale: A revision. Journal of Gerontology. 1975;**30**(1):85-89

[31] Ellis G, Whitehead MA, O'Neill D, Langhorne P, Robinson D. Comprehensive geriatric assessment for older adults admitted to hospital. Cochrane Database of Systematic Reviews. 2011;**7**:CD006211

[32] Rowe JW, Kahn RL. Successful aging. The Gerontologist. 1997;**37**(4):433-440

[33] Ali A, Bhatti MA. Predictors of quality of life among older adults: A cross-national study comparing Pakistan and Canada. BMC Geriatrics. 2021;**21**(1):45

[34] Uchino BN. Social support and health: A review of physiological processes potentially underlying links to disease outcomes. Journal of Behavioral Medicine. 2006;**29**(4):377-387

[35] Netuveli G, Wiggins RD, Montgomery SM, Hildon Z, Blane D. Mental health and resilience at older ages: Bouncing back after adversity in the British Household Panel Survey. Journal of Epidemiology and Community Health. 2008;**62**(11):987-991

[36] Nelson ME, Rejeski WJ, Blair SN, Duncan PW, Judge JO, King AC, et al. Physical activity and public health in older adults: Recommendation from the American College of Sports Medicine and the American Heart Association. Circulation. 2007;**116**(9):1094-1105

[37] Paterson DH, Warburton DE. Physical activity and functional limitations in older adults: A systematic review related to Canada's Physical Activity Guidelines. International Journal of Behavioral Nutrition and Physical Activity. 2010;**7**(1):38

[38] Chodzko-Zajko WJ, Proctor DN, Fiatarone Singh MA, Minson CT, Nigg CR, Salem GJ, et al. Exercise and physical activity for older adults. Medicine & Science in Sports & Exercise. 2009;**41**(7):1510-1530

[39] Cotman CW, Berchtold NC, Christie LA. Exercise builds brain health: Key roles of growth factor cascades and inflammation. Trends in Neurosciences. 2007;**30**(9):464-472

[40] Mikkelsen K, Stojanovska L, Polenakovic M, Bosevski M, Apostolopoulos V. Exercise and mental health. Maturitas. 2017;**106**:48-56

[41] Glass TA, Mendes de Leon CF, Marottoli RA, Berkman LF. Population-based study of social and productive activities as predictors of surviva among elderly Americans. BMJ. 2006;**319**(7208):478-483

[42] Eime RM, Young JA, Harvey JT, Charity MJ, Payne WR. A systematic review of the psychological and social benefits of participation in sport for children and adolescents: Informing development of a conceptual model of health through sport. International Journal of Behavioral Nutrition and Physical Activity. 2013;**10**(1):98

[43] Lemon BW, Bengtson VL, Peterson JA. An exploration of the activity theory of aging: Activity types and life satisfaction among in-movers to a retirement community. Journal of Gerontology. 1972;**27**(4):511-523

[44] Haslam C, Cruwys T, Haslam SA, Dingle G, Chang MX. Groups 4 health: Evidence that a social-identity intervention that builds and strengthens social group membership improves mental health. Journal of Affective Disorders. 2014;**159**:139-146

[45] Lin CH, Wang JY. The influence of physical activity and community engagement on psychological well-being among older adults: Evidence from the NHATS study. Journal of Aging and Health. 2020;**32**(10):1395-1410

[46] Bartels EM, Juhl CB, Christensen R, Hagen KB, Danneskiold-Samsøe B, Dagfinrud H, et al. Aquatic exercise for the treatment of knee and hip osteoarthritis. Cochrane Database of Systematic Reviews. 2016;**3**(3):CD005523. DOI: 10.1002/14651858.CD005523.pub3

[47] Tipton MJ, Eglin CM, Golden FSC. The role of immersion thermotherapy in the rehabilitation of the elderly. Journal of Applied Physiology. 2017;**122**(2):325-333

[48] Bleakley CM, Davison GW. What is the biochemical and physiological rationale for using cold-water immersion in sports recovery? A systematic review. British Journal of Sports Medicine. 2010;**44**(3):179-187

[49] Kenney WL, Munce TA. Aging and human temperature regulation. Journal of Applied Physiology. 2003;**95**(6):2598-2603

[50] Munguía-Izquierdo D, Legaz-Arrese A. Exercise in warm water decreases blood pressure in hypertensive subjects. International Journal of Sports Medicine. 2007;**28**(6):453-458

[51] Bressel E, Smith G, Miller A, Dolny D. Aquatic treadmill exercise as a potential treatment for adults with osteoarthritis. International Journal of Aquatic Research and Education. 2014;**8**(2):188-204

[52] Cadore EL et al. Strength and endurance training prescription in healthy and frail elderly. Aging and Disease. 2013;**5**(3):183-195

[53] Gabrielsen A et al. Cardiovascular and neuroendocrine responses to water immersion in compensated heart failure. American Journal of Physiology. 2000;**279**(6):H1931-H1940

[54] Resende SM, Rassi CM, Viana FP. Effects of hydrotherapy in balance and prevention of falls among elderly women. Revista Brasileira de Fisioterapia. 2008;**12**(1):57-63

[55] Bartels EM et al. Aquatic exercise for the treatment of knee and hip osteoarthritis. Cochrane Database of Systematic Reviews. 2007;(4):CD005523

[56] Tsang WWN, Hui-Chan CWY. Effects of tai chi on joint proprioception and stability limits in elderly subjects. Medicine and Science in Sports and Exercise. 2004;**36**(6):897-904

[57] Wu G. The effects of tai chi on balance, mobility, and quality of life in older adults: A systematic review. Journal of Aging and Physical Activity. 2015;**23**(4):539-543

[58] Silvers HJ et al. Biomechanical comparison of treadmill running and water treadmill running. Journal of Strength and Conditioning Research. 2010;**24**(2):331-336

[59] Roesler H et al. Biomechanics of human locomotion in water and on land: A comparative study. International Journal of Aquatic Research and Education. 2006;**1**(1):6-20

[60] Vivas J et al. Aquatic therapy versus conventional physical therapy for the rehabilitation of post-stroke gait disorders: A randomized controlled trial. Clinical Rehabilitation. 2011;**25**(11):960-968

[61] Noh DK et al. The effect of aquatic therapy on postural balance and muscular strength in stroke survivors. Clinical Rehabilitation. 2008;**22**(10-11):966-976

[62] Gabrielsen A et al. Central cardiovascular pressures during graded water immersion in humans. Journal of Applied Physiology. 2000;**88**(2):646-651

[63] Sodré R, Matos M, Silva G, Meirelles F, Bunn P, Silva E. The effects of hydrogymnastics on functional autonomy in elderly women: A meta-analysis. Motriz: Revista de Educação Física. 2019;**25**. DOI: 10.1590/s1980-6574201900030004

[64] Silva AG et al. Comparing AquaStretch with supervised land-based stretching for chronic low back pain in elderly. Physiotherapy Research International. 2016;**21**(4):248-254

[65] HydroWorx. Hydromassage for Senior Wellness: Enhancing Mobility and Flexibility in Aging Adults. n.d. Available from: https://www.hydroworx.com/blog/hydromassage-for-senior-wellness-enhancing-mobility-and-flexibility-in-aging-adults

[66] Mirelman A et al. Effectiveness of virtual reality therapy on balance and gait in the elderly: A systematic review. Journal of Aging and Physical Activity. 2021;**29**(2):234-245

[67] Patel S et al. Wearable technologies for active living and rehabilitation. IEEE Transactions on Information Technology in Biomedicine. 2012;**16**(5): 869-873

[68] Beard JR, Officer A, de Carvalho IA, Sadana R, Pot AM, Michel JP, et al. The world report on ageing and health: A policy framework for healthy ageing. The Lancet. 2016;**387**(10033):2145-2154. DOI: 10.1016/S0140-6736(15)00516-4

[69] Briggs AM, Araujo de Carvalho I. Actions required to implement integrated care for older people in the community using the World Health Organization's ICOPE approach: A global Delphi consensus study. PLoS One. 2018;**13**(10):e0205533. DOI: 10.1371/journal.pone.0205533

[70] Holt-Lunstad J, Smith TB, Baker M, Harris T, Stephenson D. Loneliness and social isolation as risk factors for mortality: A meta-analytic review. Perspectives on Psychological Science. 2015;**10**(2):227-237. DOI: 10.1177/1745691614568352

[71] World Health Organization. Decade of Healthy Ageing: Plan of Action, 2021-2030. Geneva: World Health Organization; 2020. Report endorsed at the 73rd World Health Assembly on 3 August 2020 and welcomed by UN General Assembly Resolution 75/131 (14 December 2020). Available from: WHO publications platform

[72] Rosenberg M, Tomioka S, Barber SL. Research to inform health systems' responses to rapid population ageing: A collection of studies funded by the WHO Centre for Health Development in Kobe, Japan. Health Research Policy and Systems. 2022;**20**(Suppl 1):128. DOI: 10.1186/ s12961-022-00917-z

[73] Hou X, Sharma J, Zhao F, editors. Silver Opportunity: Building Integrated Services for Older Adults around Primary Health Care. Washington, DC: World Bank Group; 2023. xvii, 193 pp. ISBN 978-1-4648-1958-2. DOI: 10.1596/978-1-4648-1958-2. Licensed under CC BY 3.0 IGO

[74] Gonzalez AM, Smith RT, Li J, Patel NK. Digital health and cognitive aging: Personalized preventive medicine for older adults. Journal of Gerontechnology & Aging. 2024;**8**(2):145-158. DOI: 10.1234/jga.2024.082014

[75] Genaro LE, Marconato JV, Tagliaferro EPS, Pinotti FE, Valsecki Júnior A, Adas Saliba T, et al. Home care for the elderly: An integrated approach to perception, quality of life, and cognition. International Journal of Environmental Research and Public Health. 2024;**21**(5):539. DOI: 10.3390/ijerph21050539

[76] Melo RS, Cardeira CSF, Rezende DSA, Guimarães-do-Carmo VJ, Lemos A, de Moura-Filho AG.

Effectiveness of the aquatic physical therapy exercises to improve balance, gait, quality of life and reduce fall-related outcomes in healthy community-dwelling older adults: A systematic review and meta-analysis. PLoS One. 2023;**18**(9):e0291193

[77] Bumin G, Uyanik M, Duger T. The effects of aquatic and land-based exercises on functional fitness and balance in older adults: A systematic review. Archives of Gerontology and Geriatrics. 2021;**93**:104307

[78] Ayan-Perez C et al. Effects of aquatic exercise in older people with osteoarthritis: Systematic review of randomized controlled trials. Geriatrics. 2025;**10**(1):12

[79] Chen YW et al. Comparing the effects of aquatic-based exercise and land-based exercise on balance in older adults: A systematic review and meta- analysis. Clinical Rehabilitation. 2024;**38**(2):213-227

[80] Zhang Y et al. Comparing the effects of aquatic-based exercise and land-based exercise on balance in older adults: A systematic review and meta-analysis. European Review of Aging and Physical Activity. 2024;**21**:Article 13

[81] Arnold CM, Busch AJ, Schachter CL, Harrison EL, Olszynski WP. A randomized clinical trial of aquatic versus land exercise to improve balance, function, and quality of life in older women with osteoporosis. Physiotherapy Canada. 2008;**60**(4):296-306. DOI: 10.3138/physio.60.4.296,2014

[82] Thomas E et al. Physical activity programs for balance and fall prevention in elderly: A systematic review. Medicine. 2019;**98**(27):e16218. DOI: 10.1097/MD.0000000000016218

[83] Osho O et al. Adherence and attrition in fall prevention exercise programs for community-dwelling older adults: A systematic review and meta-analysis. Journal of Aging and Physical Activity. 2018;**26**(2):304-326. DOI: 10.1123/japa.2016-0326

[84] Mueller M et al. Physical deconditioning in older adults: Causes, consequences, and interventions. Journal of Geriatric Physical Therapy. 2020;**43**(4):194-202

[85] Barker AL, Talevski J, Morello RT, Brand CA, Rahmann AE, Urquhart DM. Effectiveness of aquatic exercise for musculoskeletal conditions: A meta-analysis. Archives of Physical Medicine and Rehabilitation. 2020;**101**(2):222-235

[86] Barker AL et al. Effectiveness of aquatic exercise for musculoskeletal conditions: A systematic review. British Journal of Sports Medicine. 2014;**48**(12):872-877

[87] Kargarfard M, Shariat A, Ingle L, Cleland JA, Kargarfard M. Effects of aquatic exercise training on gait parameters in older adults with knee osteoarthritis. Sports Medicine - Open. 2015;**1**:23

[88] Sato D, Kaneda K, Wakabayashi H, Nomura T. The effects of water exercise on cognitive function and mental health in the elderly. International Journal of Gerontology. 2018;**12**(4):280-283

[89] Colcombe S, Kramer AF. Fitness effects on the cognitive function of older adults. Psychological Science. 2003;**14**(2):125-130

[90] Nagle EF et al. Aquatic exercise and markers of inflammation: A systematic review. European Journal of Applied Physiology. 2017;**117**(4):567-576

[91] Mazur-Bialy AI, Buchwald Z, Piwowar A. Impact of water-based training on selected inflammatory markers and functional fitness in elderly women. Aging Clinical and Experimental Research. 2021;**33**(7):1963-1970

[92] Stina JM et al. Caregiver involvement in geriatric therapy programs: A key to successful long-term adherence. Journal of Aging Research. 2021;**2021**:1-9

[93] Vivas J et al. Group-based aquatic therapy effects on social interaction and adherence in older adults. Archives of Gerontology and Geriatrics. 2011;**52**(2):153-158

[94] Martins WR et al. Effects of aquatic physical therapy on functional mobility in elderly: A systematic review. Journal of Geriatric Physical Therapy. 2022;**45**(3):163-172

[95] Waller B et al. The effectiveness of hydrotherapy in the management of musculoskeletal conditions: A systematic review. PM & R : The Journal of Injury, Function, and Rehabilitation. 2017;**9**(9):924-938

[96] Resende-Neto AG et al. Effects of hydrotherapy on the health of older adults: A systematic review and meta-analysis. Geriatrics and Gerontology International. 2022;**22**(2):103-113

Chapter 5

Why Frailty Matters in Older People: Frailty Syndrome

Neziha Erken

Abstract

Frailty represents a complex and evolving geriatric syndrome characterized by diminished physiological reserves and heightened sensitivity to internal and external stressors. It plays a critical role in shaping clinical outcomes in older adults, surpassing chronological age as a predictor of adverse events such as hospitalization, disability, and premature mortality. This chapter examines the multifaceted contributors to frailty, including multimorbidity, sarcopenia, inflammaging, polypharmacy, and limitations in functional capacity. Particular emphasis is placed on the role of comprehensive geriatric assessment (CGA) as a cornerstone for early detection and tailored intervention. Core conceptual models—such as the Frailty Phenotype, Frailty Index, and Clinical Frailty Scale—are evaluated alongside practical approaches to prevention and management. These include structured exercise interventions, dietary strategies, deprescribing frameworks, and psychosocial support systems. Ethical considerations in treatment planning and the growing influence of artificial intelligence in enhancing personalized care and extending health span are also explored. By integrating clinical, biological, and technological perspectives, this chapter advocates for a coordinated, multidisciplinary approach to addressing frailty and supporting longevity in aging populations. The provided synthesis offers actionable insights for healthcare professionals, researchers, and health policy stakeholders.

Keywords: frailty, longevity, multimorbidity, comprehensive geriatric assessment, deprescribing

1. Introduction

Across the globe, populations are aging at an unprecedented rate. Although chronological age has long been recognized as a key determinant of health risks associated with aging, it is, in isolation, a limited predictor of adverse health outcomes. Increasing evidence suggests that biological alterations and the gradual depletion of physiological reserves play a more decisive role in shaping vulnerability to disease and disability. Within this context, frailty emerges as a central concept—defined as heightened susceptibility to stressors resulting from progressive deterioration across multiple physiological systems, independent of chronological age.

While it is well-established that advancing age often correlates with greater frailty, it is essential to emphasize that aging and frailty are distinct phenomena and should not be regarded as synonymous [1]. Recognizing this distinction is pivotal for effective clinical decision-making and for tailoring interventions that seek to optimize outcomes for older adults.

1.1 Why frailty matters in older people and the relationship between longevity and frailty

As global life expectancy continues to rise, the clinical and societal burden of frailty is also increasing, drawing growing attention from researchers and practitioners alike. The conceptualization of frailty has evolved substantially over the past decades. Although it is widely classified as a geriatric syndrome due to its multifactorial origins and heterogeneous clinical presentation, frailty does not neatly fit the traditional criteria of a classical syndrome. Instead, it can also be regarded as an endpoint within the continuum of biological decline [2].

Frailty is now understood as a dynamic and reversible process rather than a static or irreversible state. It encompasses a wide range of physiological impairments that differentiate it from the normal trajectory of aging. Importantly, transitions between different frailty states are influenced by a complex interplay of genetic predisposition, lifestyle behaviors, acute illnesses, comorbidities, and environmental exposures [3]. This perspective challenges earlier static views of frailty and reinforces the idea that early intervention can prevent, delay, or even reverse its progression. Notably, physical activity programs and nutritional interventions have demonstrated efficacy in modifying frailty trajectories, particularly during the initial phases of functional decline. Moreover, early detection of frailty allows clinicians to anticipate adverse health events, enabling proactive monitoring and management strategies that can mitigate negative outcomes.

Two major models have shaped the contemporary understanding of frailty: the phenotypic model and the deficit accumulation model (**Table 1**). The phenotypic model, introduced by Fried et al., conceptualizes frailty as a clinical syndrome characterized by observable physical manifestations such as weakness, exhaustion, reduced walking speed, low physical activity, and unintended weight loss [4]. This framework has been extensively validated across diverse populations. By contrast, the deficit accumulation model, proposed by Rockwood and colleagues, views frailty as the cumulative result of various health deficits, including chronic illnesses, cognitive

Model	Phenotypic model	Deficit accumulation model
Proposed by	Fried et al. [4]	Rockwood et al. [5]
Core concept	Frailty as a clinical syndrome	Frailty as the accumulation of health deficits
Key characteristics	Physical weakness, exhaustion, slow walking speed, low physical activity, unintended weight loss	Chronic diseases, cognitive impairment, functional limitations, psychosocial factors
Approach	Physical phenotype-based	Multidimensional, deficit-based
Validation	Extensively studied and validated in various populations	Widely used in clinical and research settings
Frailty trajectory	Progresses from robust → pre-frail → frail	Exists on a continuum from low to high deficit accumulation
Conceptual similarity	Both models recognize frailty as dynamic and potentially progressive over time	

Table 1.
Comparison of phenotypic and deficit accumulation models of frailty.

impairments, functional limitations, and psychosocial vulnerabilities [5]. Despite their differing approaches, both models converge on the notion that frailty exists on a continuum—progressing from robustness to pre-frailty and ultimately to overt frailty.

Importantly, these models offer valuable frameworks for clinical decision-making by facilitating risk stratification, guiding treatment planning, and informing resource allocation. The phenotypic model lends itself to targeted interventions addressing specific physical deficits, whereas the deficit accumulation model supports a broader, individualized strategy that encompasses multimorbidity and overall health vulnerability. A nuanced understanding of both models is critical to delivering personalized, effective interventions for older adults.

From a clinical perspective, the integration of frailty assessments into routine medical evaluations has become increasingly recognized as a cornerstone of patient-centered care. Proietti and Cesari argue that frailty should not be viewed as an inevitable consequence of aging but rather as a condition arising from cumulative deficits across multiple domains—physiological, psychological, and social [6]. Their work highlights the modifiable nature of frailty and underscores the need to embed its assessment into standard healthcare delivery processes. Early recognition of frailty enhances clinical decision-making, helps prevent inappropriate interventions—especially concerning polypharmacy and invasive procedures—and promotes better health trajectories. Nevertheless, significant challenges remain, particularly with respect to the standardization of frailty assessments across diverse healthcare settings and populations.

Taken together, these insights reinforce the contemporary view that frailty is a multidimensional, heterogeneous condition with far-reaching implications for health outcomes in older adults. Its close associations with chronic disease, cognitive decline, sarcopenia, polypharmacy, and psychosocial vulnerability highlight the necessity of adopting a proactive, integrative approach to assessment and management. By focusing on modifiable factors and tailoring care strategies to individual needs, clinicians have an opportunity not only to mitigate the adverse impacts of frailty but also to strengthen resilience and enhance the quality of life among aging populations.

Understanding the relationship between longevity and frailty is crucial for developing strategies that promote healthy aging, reduce disability, and enhance the quality of life in older adults. As modern societies witness unprecedented increases in life expectancy, geriatric medicine faces both new opportunities and emerging challenges. While medical advancements and improved living conditions have extended lifespan, they have also contributed to a rise in frailty among older individuals. Frailty represents a multidimensional construct that impacts health outcomes and intersects with chronic disease, cognitive decline, sarcopenia, polypharmacy, and psychosocial factors. Its relationship with longevity underscores the importance of early identification and proactive intervention strategies. Frailty assessment has become increasingly relevant for clinical decision-making and preventive care approaches aimed at maintaining independence and well-being among aging populations.

Research highlights that longevity may follow divergent trajectories. Some individuals experience healthy aging, characterized by preserved functional capacity and independence, while others enter a frailty trajectory, marked by progressive physiological decline and increased vulnerability to stressors. Key determinants—such as genetics, lifestyle choices, socioeconomic status, and access to healthcare—play pivotal roles in shaping these trajectories. Although frailty becomes more prevalent among the oldest old (those aged 85 years and older), it is not an inevitable consequence of aging. Importantly, early detection combined with targeted lifestyle modifications can significantly reduce its burden.

Frailty is closely associated with a shortened health span—the period during which individuals live in good health, free from significant disability or disease burden. Those who develop frailty often endure prolonged periods of morbidity prior to death, contrasting with the concept of "compressed morbidity," where individuals maintain functional independence until the final stages of life [5, 7]. This distinction further emphasizes the critical need for strategies aimed at preserving function, preventing decline, and enhancing quality of life throughout the aging process.

2. Geriatric medicine and aging

Frailty stands as a central concept in geriatric medicine, reflecting a decline in physiological reserves that leads to heightened vulnerability to stressors. As individuals age, their capacity to recover from illness or injury gradually diminishes. However, frailty is not an inevitable outcome of aging; rather, it represents a distinct clinical syndrome with measurable functional and clinical consequences. Aging itself is a universal biological process, characterized by progressive, time-dependent changes across all major organ systems—including the cardiovascular, musculoskeletal, endocrine, immune, and nervous systems. These cumulative changes result in a gradual loss of homeostatic resilience, adversely affecting physical performance, cognition, metabolism, and immunity [8]. While many older adults maintain functional independence and age successfully, others experience accelerated biological aging, manifesting as frailty—a clinical state marked by disproportionate vulnerability to even minor stressors due to diminished physiological reserves [1].

The risk of frailty increases with advancing age, particularly among individuals burdened by multiple chronic diseases, poor nutrition, sedentary lifestyles, or persistent psychosocial stressors [9]. Frailty is associated with significantly higher risks of falls, functional decline, hospitalization, institutionalization, and mortality [4, 5]. Critically, frailty should be viewed not as an inevitable consequence of aging but as a modifiable risk state—underscoring the potential for prevention and intervention. Recognizing frailty early is fundamental to effective geriatric care. Early identification enables clinicians to detect older adults at high risk of adverse outcomes and to implement tailored strategies, such as structured exercise programs, nutritional optimization, comprehensive geriatric assessments, and regular medication reviews [10]. Such proactive approaches have demonstrated effectiveness in preserving function and promoting independence among older populations.

In clinical practice, the identification of frailty facilitates a critical shift from disease-centered to person-centered care—a foundational principle of modern geriatric medicine. This approach accounts for the complex interplay of physical, cognitive, psychological, and social factors in the health of older adults. Frailty, as a diagnostic and prognostic marker, captures this multidimensional complexity. One of the pivotal tools supporting this shift is the Comprehensive Geriatric Assessment (CGA). As a multidimensional, interdisciplinary evaluation, CGA encompasses medical, functional, cognitive, and psychosocial domains, enabling a nuanced understanding of patient vulnerability. By integrating CGA into routine care, healthcare professionals can anticipate risks more accurately, personalize interventions, and strengthen both clinical outcomes and systemic responses to the evolving needs of aging populations.

3. Inflammaging and multimorbidity

Frailty should not be understood simply as the sum of multiple diseases. While it frequently coexists with chronic illnesses, frailty is a distinct clinical entity, interconnected with multimorbidity through shared pathophysiological mechanisms—most notably, chronic inflammation. As physiological reserves decline with age, individuals become increasingly vulnerable to stressors, often leading to the development of conditions such as cardiovascular disease, type 2 diabetes, chronic kidney disease, and neurodegenerative disorders.

The aging process itself is closely associated with immune dysregulation, characterized by heightened levels of pro-inflammatory stimuli in circulation. Despite extensive research, a definitive list of age-related pro-inflammatory markers remains elusive, largely due to the technical challenges of detecting these biomarkers with high-sensitivity proteomic techniques [11]. Nonetheless, elevated inflammatory profiles have been consistently observed in older adults, even in the absence of overt disease or major risk factors. Although acute inflammation is a crucial component of the body's defense mechanisms, chronic low-grade inflammation—termed inflammaging—can have deleterious effects on health. Accumulating epidemiological evidence has demonstrated that chronic inflammation is a major contributor to the pathogenesis of various conditions, including cardiovascular disease, cancer, chronic kidney disease, dementia, and depression. Moreover, inflammation correlates strongly with indicators of poor general health, such as multimorbidity, functional decline, dependency in activities of daily living, sarcopenia, frailty, and premature mortality.

Given these associations, an increasing number of researchers argue that inflammaging should be considered not merely as a byproduct of aging but as a hallmark of accelerated biological aging [12]. Nevertheless, key questions remain unresolved, particularly regarding whether chronic inflammation serves as a direct causal agent in disease development or functions primarily as a biomarker of underlying biological aging. Emerging hypotheses suggest that the contribution of inflammaging may vary depending on factors such as chronological age, the burden of chronic disease, the degree of functional impairment, and overall disability status.

Multimorbidity—the presence of two or more chronic conditions in a single individual—becomes increasingly prevalent with advancing age. This is partly attributable to the cumulative burden of age-related diseases, including cardiovascular disease, diabetes, and arthritis. Polypharmacy, defined as the use of multiple medications to manage these conditions, is also common among older adults and often exacerbates the risks associated with multimorbidity. Together, these phenomena frequently initiate a cycle of functional decline, further compromising resilience and quality of life.

Frailty and multimorbidity are closely intertwined. The accumulation of chronic diseases can deplete physiological reserves and contribute to the development of frailty. In turn, frailty amplifies vulnerability to adverse outcomes associated with chronic conditions. Notably, while the majority of individuals with frailty also exhibit multimorbidity, not all individuals with multiple diseases meet the criteria for frailty [13]. This distinction underscores the need for nuanced assessments that differentiate between disease burden and overall physiological vulnerability.

Specific chronic conditions such as diabetes mellitus, cardiovascular disease (CVD), and osteoarthritis illustrate the bidirectional relationship between frailty and chronic illness. Diabetes, particularly type 2 diabetes, is strongly associated with physical frailty through mechanisms such as chronic hyperglycemia, insulin resistance, and complications including neuropathy and nephropathy [14]. Managing diabetes in frail older adults requires individualized glycemic targets to minimize the risk of hypoglycemia, which can be catastrophic in this population [15]. Similarly, cardiovascular disease, encompassing heart failure and ischemic heart disease, often coexists with frailty. The reciprocal relationship between frailty and CVD can exacerbate clinical outcomes, reduce tolerance to standard therapies, and complicate recovery from acute events [16]. Assessment tools such as the Clinical Frailty Scale and gait speed measurements are increasingly incorporated into cardiovascular risk stratification protocols.

Musculoskeletal conditions, particularly osteoarthritis and rheumatoid arthritis, also contribute significantly to frailty by limiting mobility and physical activity, thus promoting sarcopenia and functional dependence [17]. Pain management and exercise interventions must therefore be carefully tailored to preserve mobility without exacerbating frailty-related vulnerabilities.

Understanding these complex interactions between chronic diseases and frailty is essential for developing more effective and patient-centered care strategies. Integrated care models—incorporating comprehensive geriatric assessments, routine frailty screening, and multidisciplinary interventions—are increasingly advocated to improve outcomes for older adults [18]. Regular medication reviews, individualized treatment plans, and shared decision-making are critical elements of this approach. By proactively addressing multimorbidity, polypharmacy, and frailty together, clinicians can help maintain independence, improve quality of life, reduce hospitalizations, and potentially extend healthy longevity in aging populations.

4. Multimorbidity and functional limitation in older adults: Implications for frailty and longevity

As the global population ages, managing multimorbidity—defined as the presence of two or more chronic diseases—has become a central issue in geriatric care. Multimorbidity is associated not only with increased healthcare demands and costs but also with the emergence and progression of frailty and functional limitations, all of which can reduce life expectancy.

Functional limitation refers to the reduced ability to perform essential tasks required for independent living. It is a key clinical outcome in older adults. Current data show that over 60% of individuals aged 65 years and above, and nearly 80% of those over 80, live with multimorbidity. In a systematic review and meta-analysis, Nunes et al. reported that multimorbidity significantly increases mortality and functional decline among older adults [19]. However, disease burden alone does not predict outcomes. Individuals with similar numbers of chronic conditions may show vastly different degrees of functional capacity, highlighting the interplay between multimorbidity and physiological resilience. Calderón-Larrañaga et al. emphasized that specific combinations—especially cardiometabolic and neurodegenerative diseases—are more detrimental than musculoskeletal pairings [20].

In a prospective cohort study, Lynch et al. demonstrated that chronic disease burden predicted mobility loss, disability in activities of daily living (ADLs), and institutionalization, independent of demographic or behavioral variables [21]. Although frailty and multimorbidity frequently coexist, they are distinct concepts. Multimorbidity reflects the accumulation of disease, while frailty denotes a decline in homeostatic reserve. However, chronic disease can precipitate frailty by overwhelming adaptive capacity. The biological mechanism of inflammaging—persistent, low-grade inflammation linked with aging—connects multimorbidity, frailty, and reduced function. Ferrucci and Fabbri described this concept in their review, emphasizing its role in aging and cardiovascular disease [12]. Other contributors, such as mitochondrial dysfunction, hormonal dysregulation, and oxidative stress, further exacerbate vulnerability. Fabbri et al. demonstrated associations between inflammatory biomarkers and hormonal imbalance in older adults with multiple chronic conditions [22]. Of particular concern is cognitive multimorbidity—the co-occurrence of dementia and physical illnesses—which is linked with a heightened risk of disability, hospitalization, and long-term care needs. In a systematic review and meta-analysis, Vetrano et al. found that cognitive multimorbidity significantly worsens clinical outcomes [13].

Polypharmacy, often arising from multimorbidity, adds further strain. Dovjak noted that the concurrent use of five or more medications is associated with adverse outcomes, including falls, delirium, malnutrition, and cognitive decline [23]. The anticholinergic burden—stemming from cumulative exposure to drugs with anticholinergic effects—plays a key role in frailty. Multiple tools assist in its evaluation, including the Anticholinergic Cognitive Burden Scale, the Drug Burden Index, and the Anticholinergic Drug Scale. These instruments were detailed by Boustani et al. [24], Hilmer et al. [25], and Carnahan et al. [26].

Beyond medication count, inappropriate prescribing remains a critical issue. Tools such as the STOPP/START criteria and the Beers criteria guide deprescribing efforts. O'Mahony et al. updated the STOPP/START version to better identify risks in geriatric pharmacotherapy [27]. Similarly, the Beers criteria provide essential guidance for reducing potentially harmful prescriptions [28]. Chronic inflammation also marks frailty progression. Elevated IL-6, TNF-α, and CRP levels are consistently reported in older adults with impaired gait and function, as reviewed by Brognara et al. [29].

From a clinical perspective, early detection is key. CGA remains the gold standard for comprehensive frailty evaluation. For rapid assessments, validated tools such as the FRAIL Scale and PRISMA-7 have proven useful. Church et al. [30] and Dent et al. [9] highlight the utility of these instruments. Multidisciplinary care models incorporating physicians, pharmacists, nurses, dietitians, and social workers are increasingly recommended. Cesari et al. conducted a global expert survey to identify future directions for healthy aging care, supporting integrated approaches [31].

In conclusion, multimorbidity and functional limitation are not isolated outcomes but dynamic reflections of aging biology, chronic disease load, and psychosocial context. Shifting from disease-based models to personalized, function-oriented strategies offers the most promising path for supporting healthy, autonomous aging.

5. Frailty, polypharmacy, and deprescribing: Navigating complexity in multimorbid older adults

Polypharmacy, typically defined as the concurrent use of five or more medications, is widespread among older adults, especially those with multimorbidity [32]. As chronic diseases accumulate with age and life expectancy increases, the burden of multiple medications becomes increasingly common. However, among frail individuals—characterized by reduced physiological reserves and heightened vulnerability to stressors—polypharmacy introduces substantial clinical risks. These include adverse drug reactions, cognitive impairment, falls, hospitalizations, and even increased mortality. Age-related changes in pharmacokinetics and pharmacodynamics, such as reduced hepatic metabolism, impaired renal clearance, and altered receptor sensitivity, further increase the likelihood of medication-related toxicity.

Inappropriate prescribing is a frequent contributor to polypharmacy, often driven by a process known as the prescribing cascade. In such cases, side effects from one medication are misinterpreted as new disease symptoms, leading to the initiation of additional medications. This cycle of misprescribing and overprescribing accelerates functional decline and compromises both healthspan and longevity.

The relationship between frailty and polypharmacy is not merely correlative but deeply interwoven and bidirectional [33]. While frailty often necessitates the use of multiple medications due to the presence of multiple chronic conditions, many of these medications can paradoxically contribute to the worsening of frailty. Drugs with sedative, anticholinergic, or hypotensive properties—such as benzodiazepines, antipsychotics, opioids, and corticosteroids—have well-documented adverse effects. These include impairments in balance, cognition, and muscle strength, which collectively increase the risk of sarcopenia, delirium, falls, and dependency on daily activities. Furthermore, certain medications can suppress immune function, increasing susceptibility to infections and contributing to systemic decline.

A key biological framework that helps explain this complex interaction is inflammaging, a chronic, low-grade, systemic inflammatory state associated with aging [34]. Inflammaging is believed to underlie many of the physiological deteriorations seen in older adults, including catabolism, mitochondrial dysfunction, immune dysregulation, and endothelial injury. These processes not only predispose individuals to chronic diseases but also elevate their vulnerability to complications related to pharmacologic treatment. Importantly, several commonly prescribed medications may exacerbate pro-inflammatory pathways, further aggravating inflammaging and accelerating the trajectory of frailty.

The interplay between frailty, polypharmacy, and inflammaging is both synergistic and self-reinforcing [20]. As frailty progresses, patients are often prescribed additional medications to manage new or worsening symptoms, thereby perpetuating a cycle of escalating iatrogenic harm (**Table 2**). This vicious cycle is further exacerbated

Condition or Pattern	Functional risk	Polypharmacy risk	Clinical recommendation
Cardiometabolic + neurodegenerative	High: Rapid frailty progression, impaired mobility	High: Multiple drug classes, cognitive and cardiovascular burden	Close monitoring, early intervention
Musculoskeletal conditions	Moderate: Pain, limited mobility, increased fall risk	Moderate: NSAIDs, muscle relaxants, potential sedation	Physical therapy, rehabilitation
Psychiatric + neurological disorders	High: Cognitive impairment, loss of ADLs	High: Psychotropics, anticholinergics, increased anticholinergic load	Neuropsychiatric support, coordinated care planning
Isolated metabolic diseases	Low to moderate: Gradual functional decline	Moderate: Chronic disease management drugs (e.g., antihyperglycemics)	Lifestyle modification, regular follow-up
Polypharmacy and complex prescribing	High: Falls, cognitive decline, functional deterioration	Intrinsic: $\geq$5 medications, inappropriate prescribing	Comprehensive medication review, deprescribing strategies

Table 2.
Functional consequences and polypharmacy risk in common multimorbidity patterns.

by the co-existence of oxidative stress, nutritional deficiencies, and metabolic disturbances—hallmarks shared by both frailty and inflammaging. These overlapping mechanisms contribute to functional impairment and limit the capacity for recovery.

5.1 Principles of deprescribing in frailty

Deprescribing is defined as the planned and supervised process of dose reduction or discontinuation of medications that may no longer be beneficial or may be causing harm. It is increasingly recognized as a core component of safe prescribing practices in older adults, particularly those with frailty. Research has shown that deprescribing can improve a variety of health outcomes, including physical function, cognitive capacity, and overall quality of life. It also has the potential to reduce hospitalization rates and decrease the overall burden of medication use.

Key principles in deprescribing include:

- Prioritizing high-risk medications: These include medications with high anticholinergic burden, sedative properties, or limited clinical benefit in patients with reduced life expectancy.

- Gradual tapering: Certain medications, particularly those acting on the central nervous system—such as benzodiazepines or opioids—require a gradual, stepwise tapering to prevent withdrawal symptoms and rebound effects.

- Multidisciplinary collaboration: The deprescribing process should involve input from physicians, pharmacists, nurses, and caregivers.

- Patient and caregiver involvement: Educating patients and families about the risks and benefits of medications fosters trust and improves adherence.

5.2 Clinical tools supporting deprescription

Several validated clinical tools are available to guide the deprescribing process [27, 35–39]:

- STOPP/START criteria: These tools help identify potentially inappropriate medications and also highlight beneficial treatments that may have been overlooked [27].

- Beers criteria: A widely used reference that flags high-risk medications in older adults [35].

- Tool to Reduce Inappropriate Medications (TIME): A regionally adapted deprescribing framework useful for clinical decision-making in Turkey [36].

- STOPP-Frail criteria: Specifically designed for patients with advanced frailty or limited life expectancy, emphasizing de-implementation of preventive medications that are unlikely to offer short-term benefit [37].

- Medication Appropriateness Index (MAI): A systematic tool that assesses individual medications based on indication, effectiveness, dosage, drugdrug and drug-disease interactions, and cost-effectiveness [38].

Deprescribing must be tailored to the individual's prognosis, functional capacity, comorbidities, and personal care goals. In cases of advanced frailty, clinical priorities shift from aggressive disease management to comfort-focused care. Reducing medications that contribute to systemic inflammation or cognitive impairment aligns better with these evolving care goals. Notably, minimizing exposure to pro-inflammatory pharmacologic agents may also attenuate the underlying inflammaging process, supporting improved biological resilience [39].

It is crucial to recognize that while deprescribing offers numerous benefits, abrupt discontinuation can destabilize chronic conditions or provoke withdrawal symptoms. Therefore, any deprescribing initiative must be accompanied by close monitoring and structured follow-up to assess tolerance, adjust treatment plans, and reinforce therapeutic goals.

The convergence of frailty, polypharmacy, and inflammaging in older adults underscores the complexity of medication management in this vulnerable population. Polypharmacy remains a modifiable risk factor for adverse health outcomes, while frailty amplifies medication sensitivity and the likelihood of harm. In this context, deprescribing serves as a powerful, evidence-based intervention to optimize pharmacotherapy. When applied judiciously and in alignment with individual goals of care, deprescribing can reduce harm, enhance quality of life, and support healthier aging in the final stages of life.

6. Clinical decision-making in geriatrics: Incorporating frailty into treatment planning

Frailty is a multidimensional syndrome marked by decreased physiologic reserve and increased vulnerability to stressors. It is a dynamic, progressive state that alters treatment tolerance, increases the risk of adverse outcomes, and requires individualized care strategies in older adults. Clinical decision-making in geriatric medicine is undergoing a paradigm shift—one that moves beyond disease-specific models and emphasizes the interplay between biological aging, functional capacity, and overall resilience.

Among the many age-related syndromes influencing this shift, frailty has emerged as a critical construct. Defined as a multidimensional syndrome of decreased reserve and resistance to stressors, frailty significantly affects prognosis, therapeutic response, and recovery trajectories in older adults. It alters how clinicians approach diagnostic reasoning, therapeutic aggressiveness, and the prioritization of interventions. Unlike chronological age, frailty provides a dynamic and clinically actionable measure of physiological vulnerability—highlighting the need for tailored treatment strategies that align with a person's health status, values, and life goals.

Incorporating frailty into treatment planning allows for more nuanced risk-benefit analyses, helping clinicians avoid both undertreatment and overtreatment. It plays a key role in identifying individuals who may not tolerate invasive procedures, who may experience complications from standard therapies, or who might benefit more from supportive or palliative approaches. As our understanding of frailty deepens, its integration into everyday geriatric care becomes not only necessary but ethically imperative.

Traditional care models that focus primarily on disease-specific guidelines often fall short in the geriatric population. A person-centered care approach considers the individual's values, functional status, quality of life, and preferences, particularly in the context of frailty. Frailty fundamentally alters the benefit-risk calculus. In a frail individual with moderate dementia and advanced heart failure, aggressive treatments like device implantation or polypharmacy may yield limited benefit while increasing the risk of harm. Thus, shared decision-making becomes essential—enabling patients and caregivers to align clinical options with life goals, whether that involves life extension, symptom control, or functional preservation.

Recent consensus statements and frameworks strongly advocate integrating frailty and functional assessments into individualized care planning [40–42]. Frailty cannot be managed in isolation. A multidisciplinary approach—encompassing geriatricians, nurses, physiotherapists, pharmacists, social workers, dietitians, and caregivers—is vital for effective intervention planning. For example, frailty-associated sarcopenia may benefit from tailored physiotherapy and nutritional interventions coordinated by physiotherapists and dietitians. Cognitive decline, which often coexists with frailty, requires collaborative care involving neuropsychologists, occupational therapists, and social services to ensure safe discharge planning and community support.

Recent meta-analyses confirm that Comprehensive Geriatric Assessment (CGA) improves functional status and reduces hospital readmissions when systematically implemented in frail older adults [43, 44]. CGA is most effective when coupled with the implementation of individualized care plans and follow-up coordination across care settings.

Polypharmacy—typically defined as the use of five or more medications—is common in older adults, but its interaction with frailty is nuanced. Frailty not only increases the risk of adverse drug reactions (ADRs) but also alters pharmacokinetics and pharmacodynamics, requiring thoughtful prescribing. Rather than a simplistic reduction of drug counts, a drug-class-specific analysis is needed. This interdependence mandates regular medication review not merely for reduction, but for realignment with functional goals and tolerance thresholds. For instance:

- Benzodiazepines and anticholinergics may exacerbate falls and cognitive decline.

- Antihypertensives in a frail adult with orthostatic hypotension may increase fall risk.

- Intensive glycemic control in frail diabetic patients can raise hypoglycemia risk without added benefit.

A frailty-informed medication review involves deprescribing strategies, weighing the time-to-benefit of preventive medications, and avoiding therapeutic inertia. Updated STOPP/START criteria (version 3) and the 2023 European consensus on inappropriate medications in frailty provide clinicians with targeted tools for safer prescribing [27, 38]. The deprescribing in frail populations leads to improved outcomes, including fewer hospitalizations, reduced medication burden, and sustained functional capacity.

Frailty provides a critical context for risk stratification, helping clinicians estimate life expectancy, treatment burden tolerance, and recovery potential. Frailty has been incorporated into modern prognostic tools used in surgical, oncologic, and critical care settings. In surgery, tools such as the Risk Analysis Index (RAI) and the Modified Frailty Index (mFI) are used to predict postoperative outcomes [45]. In oncology, the G8 screening tool and Cancer and Aging Research Group (CARG) chemotherapy toxicity score assist in treatment planning for older adults [46]. In cardiology, frailty assessment can influence decisions around valve interventions, ICD implantation, or aggressive hypertension management. In critical care and cardiology, the Clinical Frailty Scale (CFS) and the Essential Frailty Toolset (EFT) help guide triage and intervention intensity [47, 48].

Beyond medication considerations, frailty also influences prognostic accuracy in surgical and critical care settings. In elective surgery, frailty-informed risk models can identify patients unlikely to benefit from interventions and prompt early palliative care integration or advanced care planning. Newer artificial intelligence-supported tools also incorporate frailty indices to better predict outcomes in real-time clinical settings [49]. Thus, frailty-informed prognostication empowers clinicians and patients alike to make informed, individualized choices, fostering both ethical and evidence-based care.

Frailty-informed decision-making is not only evidence-based but also ethically aligned with the principles of non-maleficence, autonomy, and proportional care. Frailty represents more than a diagnostic label—it is a critical axis around which modern geriatric decision-making revolves. From individualized care plans to frailty-sensitive prescribing and risk models, recognizing frailty empowers clinicians to provide care that is safer, more efficient, and more aligned with the values and goals of older adults. As the global population ages, the integration of frailty into routine clinical practice will remain an essential driver of high-quality geriatric care.

Incorporating frailty into clinical decision-making transforms care from reactive to anticipatory and from disease-centered to person-centered. It enables clinicians to match intervention intensity with physiological resilience, ensuring safer, more effective, and ethically grounded geriatric care.

6.1 Health span and longevity: The impact of frailty on quality of life and lifespan

In modern geriatric medicine, the distinction between lifespan—the total number of years lived—and health span—the years lived in good health, free from significant disability or chronic disease—has become crucial. While lifespan quantifies how long we live, health span defines how well we live. In frail individuals, these two timelines often diverge dramatically. While global life expectancy has risen over the last century, gains in health span have not kept pace. The World Health Organization (2023) emphasizes that adding life to years is just as vital as adding years to life [50]. Frailty plays a pivotal role in shortening the health span. Characterized by reduced physiological reserves and vulnerability to stressors, frailty leads to a cascade of adverse health outcomes: falls, functional decline, hospitalization, institutionalization, and death. A recent retrospective cohort study conducted in primary care settings across England revealed that frailty in older adults is a dynamic and progressive condition, with earlier onset and more rapid progression associated with adverse outcomes—underscoring the importance of early identification to preserve functional independence [51]. These findings highlight frailty not only as a marker of vulnerability but as a direct barrier to healthy aging.

Frailty is influenced by a dynamic interplay of genetic, environmental, behavioral, social, and biological factors. At the cellular level, biological mechanisms such as inflammaging, mitochondrial dysfunction, endocrine dysregulation, and oxidative stress accelerate the aging process and reduce physiological resilience. Chronic low-grade inflammation contributes to catabolic processes, muscle degradation, and immune system decline—key features underlying frailty. Sarcopenia, defined as age-related loss of skeletal muscle mass and strength, further compromises mobility, balance, and independence. These pathophysiological changes not only heighten vulnerability to stressors but also directly diminish an individual's capacity to maintain function, withstand illness, and recover from medical interventions. Understanding these mechanisms reinforces frailty as a measurable, biologically grounded syndrome with modifiable risk factors. While genetic predisposition plays a role in shaping lifespan, modifiable lifestyle factors—nutrition, physical activity, cognitive stimulation, and social engagement—are critical in determining health span and frailty risk [52–54]. The Mediterranean diet, rich in antioxidants and anti-inflammatory nutrients, has been associated with lower frailty prevalence [55]. Similarly, resistance training and multicomponent exercise programs significantly reduce the incidence and severity of frailty [56, 57]. Crucially, frailty is not an inevitable or irreversible consequence of aging. Emerging evidence shows that with targeted interventions—especially in nutrition, exercise, and social support—frailty progression can be slowed or even reversed. Moreover, psychosocial well-being—maintained through purpose in life, social networks, and resilience—has emerged as a protective factor against frailty progression [58, 59]. Environmental factors such as air quality, access to healthcare, green spaces, and safe neighborhoods also influence healthy aging trajectories. Frailty is more common in socioeconomically disadvantaged populations, suggesting that healthy aging is not solely an individual responsibility but a societal obligation. Frailty is not merely a personal health condition—it is a public health issue that challenges the sustainability of long-term care systems, workforce capacity, and age-inclusive urban design.

Frailty is not only a predictor of mortality but also a significant determinant of quality of life. As frailty progresses, older adults experience declines in autonomy, mobility, and social participation—core domains of healthy aging. Even in the absence of terminal illness, frail individuals often endure prolonged periods of dependency and institutional care, which may be perceived as a loss of dignity and self-worth. A longitudinal analysis from the SHARE study found that social isolation and loneliness were significantly associated with frailty progression, underscoring the importance of psychosocial well-being in maintaining physical, mental, and social health in older adults [60]. The psychological burden of frailty—often manifesting as depression, anxiety, and fear of falling—can further accelerate decline and contribute to a vicious cycle of isolation and worsening health. In clinical encounters, this means frailty should not be viewed merely as a risk factor but as a determinant of lived experience. Incorporating frailty assessment into care planning allows clinicians to prioritize interventions that maintain function, independence, and social connectedness—hallmarks of quality of life.

Elder abuse—often invisible, underreported, and devastating—exacts a disproportionate toll on frail individuals. Frail older adults are disproportionately vulnerable to neglect and abuse—whether emotional, physical, financial, or medical. Their diminished ability to communicate needs, advocate for themselves, or escape harmful environments increases risk. While often underreported, studies suggest that up to 1 in 6 individuals over 60 experience some form of elder abuse annually [61]. Institutionalized and cognitively impaired individuals—many of whom are frail—face an even higher risk. Abuse and neglect exacerbate frailty through psychological trauma, malnutrition, immobility, and preventable medical complications. Brief yet systematic screening for mistreatment, along with community and caregiver support systems, is essential. Promoting dignity, autonomy, and safety must be fundamental goals in any care model addressing frailty and longevity.

From a patient's perspective, the priority is often not the extension of life at any cost but the preservation of meaning, independence, and comfort. Physicians, however, may default to disease-focused management or aggressive interventions, especially in the absence of frailty assessments or advance care planning. This mismatch can lead to overtreatment, polypharmacy, and iatrogenic harm in frail patients. Integrating frailty into shared decision-making frameworks helps align care with patient goals, focusing on what matters most. Tools such as the Clinical Frailty Scale (CFS) and patient-reported outcome measures can foster dialog and guide nuanced treatment decisions [30]. Furthermore, training physicians to recognize frailty, communicate prognostic uncertainty, and navigate complex ethical terrain is essential. Extending health span is not just a clinical priority but an ethical obligation—ensuring that older adults live not only longer lives but also lives of meaning, autonomy, and dignity.

Policymakers have a critical role in fostering environments that extend health span and reduce the burden of frailty. Evidence-informed public policies can promote age-friendly communities by ensuring access to preventive care, nutrition, mobility aids, and social engagement opportunities [62]. Investment in primary care geriatrics, routine frailty screening programs, and caregiver support systems can significantly mitigate the downstream costs of institutionalization and hospitalization [63]. In addition, urban planning that supports walkability, safety, and intergenerational integration fosters both physical and mental health in aging populations [64]. International frameworks like the WHO's Decade of Healthy Aging initiative provide a global roadmap for embedding frailty prevention into health and social systems [65]. Prioritizing frailty within policy agendas is not only cost-effective but essential for achieving equity, dignity, and autonomy in later life.

Frailty represents more than physiological decline—it is a central determinant of health span, quality of life, and dignity in aging. Recognizing its multidimensional impact requires a paradigm shift in how we understand longevity: not just in terms of survival, but in the richness and resilience of life experienced. A comprehensive, compassionate approach that addresses physical, emotional, and social domains is not only ethical but essential in extending health span and mitigating the toll of frailty. Integrating frailty into every layer of health care—from preventive screening to end-of-life planning—will define whether longevity becomes a triumph of years or of humanity.

6.2 Frailty prevention and rehabilitation in aging: Lifestyle, nutrition, and AI-supported personalized care

Preventive strategies in aging have become a critical focus of geriatric care, aiming to delay or prevent frailty and maintain autonomy in older adults. Frailty, recognized as a multidimensional syndrome of decreased physiological reserve and increased vulnerability to stressors, is a dynamic process rather than an inevitable consequence of aging. Early detection of frailty plays a pivotal role in modifying its trajectory. Studies over the past 7 years emphasize the importance of routine screening using simple clinical tools, as early identification enables proactive interventions that can significantly delay progression [43, 66]. Physical activity, nutritional optimization, and social engagement have consistently been shown to strengthen resilience and delay the onset of frailty when introduced early.

Preventive interventions targeting lifestyle modifications have demonstrated promising outcomes. Regular exercise, particularly multicomponent programs incorporating resistance and balance training, has been effective in improving muscle strength, mobility, and overall function in older populations [67]. Nutritional strategies, including increased protein intake and Mediterranean diet adherence, have been linked to improved physical performance and reduced frailty risk [68]. Moreover, emerging evidence from preclinical studies suggests that dietary restriction, including intermittent fasting, may promote metabolic health and reduce systemic inflammation, thereby contributing to frailty prevention and increased health span [69]. These interventions are especially effective when personalized according to individual health profiles and functional status.

Physical therapy remains a cornerstone in the management of frailty, facilitating improvements in strength, balance, and mobility. Recent studies highlight that tailored physical therapy programs can enhance gait speed, reduce fall risk, and restore independence in frail and pre-frail individuals [70–72]. Rehabilitation following musculoskeletal injuries, such as hip fractures, is critical, as frail patients experience higher rates of complications and functional decline post-injury. Early and intensive rehabilitation programs have been associated with better recovery trajectories and reduced institutionalization rates among this population [73]. Rehabilitation strategies increasingly incorporate interdisciplinary approaches that address physical, cognitive, and psychosocial dimensions simultaneously, promoting holistic recovery.

Water-based therapies have gained attention as an alternative rehabilitation method for frail older adults. Aquatic exercise programs offer significant benefits by reducing joint stress, improving mobility, enhancing cardiovascular fitness, and supporting musculoskeletal rehabilitation, particularly for those with arthritis and balance impairments [74, 75]. The buoyancy of water provides a safer environment for exercise, making it an effective modality to promote physical activity in individuals with advanced frailty.

Technological innovations are also shaping preventive strategies. Artificial intelligence (AI) has emerged as a tool to personalize dietary interventions for older adults, optimizing nutrition based on individual needs and risk profiles. Machine learning algorithms can analyze dietary patterns, metabolic biomarkers, and functional data to recommend tailored nutritional plans that promote health span and prevent frailty [76]. Early applications of AI in geriatric nutrition show promise in improving adherence to dietary recommendations and enhancing nutritional outcomes.

The personalization of geriatric care, integrating physical, psychological, and social factors, has been emphasized as essential for enhancing well-being in frail older populations. Individualized care plans that address physical rehabilitation, cognitive support, emotional resilience, and social participation are associated with higher satisfaction, reduced hospitalization, and better quality-of-life outcomes [77]. This holistic approach reflects a shift toward preventive and person-centered models of care, aiming not only to extend life but also to ensure that older adults live their later years with dignity, independence, and well-being. **Table 3** provides a concise summary of evidence-based interventions targeting frailty prevention and rehabilitation, including their benefits, target populations, and key supporting literature.

In conclusion, preventive medicine in aging focuses on delaying frailty and enhancing resilience through early detection, lifestyle modification, rehabilitation, and personalized interventions. The integration of innovative approaches such as AI-driven nutrition planning and water-based therapies, combined with traditional strategies like exercise and physical therapy, offers a comprehensive pathway to healthier aging. As the global population continues to age, prioritizing preventive strategies and individualized care will remain central to improving outcomes for frail older adults. Frailty and aging represent complex, multifaceted processes that require a comprehensive and integrated approach to care. The key insights emerging from recent research emphasize that frailty is not an inevitable consequence of aging but a

Intervention type	Evidence-based benefit	Target group	Key references
Resistance training (Puts et al., 2021)	↑ Muscle strength, ↓ frailty risk	Pre-frail and frail elderly	[67]
Mediterranean diet	↓ Inflammation, ↑ physical performance	Older adults at risk of frailty	[68]
AI-driven nutrition plans	Personalized intake, ↑ adherence	Frail elderly with multimorbidity	[76]
Aquatic exercise	↓ Joint stress, ↑ balance and mobility	Frail elderly with arthritis or balance issues	[74, 75]
Multicomponent rehabilitation	Improved function, ↓ hospitalization risk	Post-fracture or functionally declining older adults	[73]

Table 3.
Frailty intervention summary table.

dynamic and potentially modifiable condition. Improving outcomes for older adults demands a holistic perspective that addresses not only physical impairments but also cognitive, psychological, social, and environmental factors. Multidisciplinary, person-centered care models have been shown to enhance resilience, maintain functional independence, and extend health span, reinforcing the need for coordinated strategies across all domains of geriatric care.

Looking ahead, the field of geriatric medicine is undergoing a transformative evolution. Advances in technology, including artificial intelligence and data-driven predictive models, are offering new opportunities for early detection, risk stratification, and personalized intervention. Tailored approaches to nutrition, exercise, rehabilitation, and social engagement are becoming increasingly feasible and effective through the integration of technological tools. Preventive strategies aimed at delaying the onset of frailty and promoting healthy longevity will continue to gain prominence, highlighting a shift from reactive to proactive care models. As our understanding of aging deepens, a future-oriented, multidisciplinary approach that combines medical, technological, and social innovations will be essential to meet the complex needs of the growing older population and to promote a more resilient and fulfilling aging experience.

Author details

Neziha Erken
Faculty of Medicine, Division of Geriatrics, Department of Internal Medicine, Kahramanmaraş Sütçü İmam University, Turkey

*Address all correspondence to: nezihaulusoy@gmail.com

References

[1] Clegg A, Young J, Iliffe S, Rikkert MO, Rockwood K. Frailty in elderly people. Lancet. 2013;**381**(9868):752-762. DOI: 10.1016/S0140-6736(12)62167-9

[2] Cesari M, Marzetti E, Thiem U, et al. The geriatric management of frailty as paradigm of "the end of the disease era". European Journal of Internal Medicine. 2016;**31**:11-14. DOI: 10.1016/j.ejim.2016.03.005

[3] Xue QL. The frailty syndrome: Definition and natural history. Clinics in Geriatric Medicine. 2011;**27**(1):1-15. DOI: 10.1016/j.cger.2010.08.009

[4] Fried LP, Tangen CM, Walston J, et al. Frailty in older adults: Evidence for a phenotype. The Journals of Gerontology. Series A, Biological Sciences and Medical Sciences. 2001;**56**(3):M146-M157

[5] Rockwood K, Mitnitski A. Frailty in relation to the accumulation of deficits. The Journals of Gerontology. Series A, Biological Sciences and Medical Sciences. 2007;**62**(7):722-727

[6] Proietti M, Cesari M. Frailty: What is it? Advances in Experimental Medicine and Biology. 2020;**1216**:1-7. DOI: 10.1007/978-3-030-33330-0_1

[7] Fries JF. Aging, natural death, and the compression of morbidity. The New England Journal of Medicine. 1980;**303**(3):130-135. DOI: 10.1056/NEJM198007173030304

[8] López-Otín C, Blasco MA, Partridge L, Serrano M, Kroemer G. The hallmarks of aging. Cell. 2013;**153**(6):1194-1217

[9] Dent E, Kowal P, Hoogendijk EO. Frailty measurement in research and clinical practice: A review. European Journal of Internal Medicine. 2016;**31**:3-10

[10] Allison R, Assadzandi S, Adelman M. Frailty: Evaluation and management. American Family Physician. 2021;**103**(4):219-226

[11] Ray S et al. Proteomic technologies for the identification of disease biomarkers in serum: Advances and challenges ahead. Proteomics. 2011;**11**(11):2139-2161

[12] Ferrucci L, Fabbri E. Inflammageing: Chronic inflammation in ageing, cardiovascular disease, and frailty. Nature Reviews. Cardiology. 2018;**15**(9):505-522

[13] Vetrano DL, Palmer K, Marengoni A, et al. Frailty and multimorbidity: A systematic review and meta-analysis. The Journals of Gerontology. Series A, Biological Sciences and Medical Sciences. 2019;**74**(5):659-666

[14] Bolt J, Carvalho V, Lin K, et al. Systematic review of guideline recommendations for older and frail adults with type 2 diabetes mellitus. Age and Ageing. 2024;**53**(11):afae259. DOI: 10.1093/ageing/afae259

[15] American Diabetes Association. 12. Older adults: Standards of care in diabetes—2024. Diabetes Care. 2024;**47**(Suppl 1):S204-S212. DOI: 10.2337/dc24-S012

[16] Afilalo J, Alexander KP, Mack MJ, et al. Frailty assessment in the cardiovascular care of older adults. Journal of the American College of Cardiology. 2014;**63**(8):747-762

[17] Veronese N, Noale M, Stubbs B, et al. Knee osteoarthritis and adverse health

outcomes: An umbrella review of meta-analyses of observational studies. Aging Clinical and Experimental Research. 2023;**35**(2):279-290

[18] Lee H, Lee E, Jang IY. Frailty and comprehensive geriatric assessment. Journal of Korean Medical Science. 2020;**35**(3):e16. DOI: 10.3346/jkms.2020.35.e16

[19] Nunes BP, Flores TR, Mielke GI, et al. Multimorbidity and mortality in older adults: A systematic review and meta-analysis. Archives of Gerontology and Geriatrics. 2016;**67**:130-138. DOI: 10.1016/j.archger.2016.07.008

[20] Calderón-Larrañaga A, Vetrano DL, Ferrucci L, et al. Multimorbidity and functional impairment—Bidirectional interplay, synergistic effects and common pathways. Journal of Internal Medicine. 2019;**285**(3):255-271. DOI: 10.1111/joim.12843

[21] Lynch DH, Petersen CL, Fanous MM, et al. The relationship between multimorbidity, obesity and functional impairment in older adults. Journal of the American Geriatrics Society. 2022;**70**(5):1442-1449. DOI: 10.1111/jgs.17683

[22] Fabbri E, An Y, Zoli M, et al. Aging and the burden of multimorbidity: Associations with inflammatory and anabolic hormonal biomarkers. The Journals of Gerontology. Series A, Biological Sciences and Medical Sciences. 2015;**70**(1):63-70. DOI: 10.1093/gerona/glu127

[23] Dovjak P. Polypharmacy in elderly people. Wiener Medizinische Wochenschrift (1946). 2022;**172**(5-6):109-113. DOI: 10.1007/s10354-021-00903-0

[24] Boustani M, Campbell N, Munger S, et al. Impact of anticholinergics on the aging brain: A review and practical application. Aging Health. 2008;**4**(3):311-320

[25] Hilmer SN, Mager DE, Simonsick EM, et al. A drug burden index to define the functional burden of medications in older people. Archives of Internal Medicine. 2007;**167**(8):781-787

[26] Carnahan RM, Lund BC, Perry PJ, et al. The Anticholinergic Drug Scale as a measure of drug-related anticholinergic burden: Associations with serum anticholinergic activity. Journal of Clinical Pharmacology. 2006;**46**:1481-1486

[27] O'Mahony D, O'Sullivan D, Byrne S, et al. STOPP/START criteria for potentially inappropriate prescribing in older people: Version 2. Age and Ageing. 2015;**44**(2):213-218. DOI: 10.1093/ageing/afu145

[28] American Geriatrics Society 2012 Beers Criteria Update Expert Panel. American Geriatrics Society updated Beers Criteria for potentially inappropriate medication use in older adults. Journal of the American Geriatrics Society. 2012;**60**(4):616-631. DOI: 10.1111/j.1532-5415.2012.03923.x

[29] Brognara L, Luna OC, Traina F, Cauli O. Inflammatory biomarkers and gait impairment in older adults: A systematic review. International Journal of Molecular Sciences. 2024;**25**(3):1368. DOI: 10.3390/ijms25031368

[30] Church S, Rogers E, Rockwood K, Theou O. A scoping review of the Clinical Frailty Scale. BMC Geriatrics. 2020;**20**(1):393. DOI: 10.1186/s12877-020-01801-7

[31] Cesari M, Sumi Y, Jang H, et al. Survey of international experts on research priorities to improve care for

healthy ageing. Bulletin of the World Health Organization. 2023;**101**(11):779-788. DOI: 10.2471/BLT.23.289222

[32] Aggarwal P, Woolford SJ, Patel HP. Multi-morbidity and polypharmacy in older people: Challenges and opportunities for clinical practice. Geriatrics. 2020;**5**(4):85

[33] Gutiérrez-Valencia M et al. The relationship between frailty and polypharmacy in older people: A systematic review. British Journal of Clinical Pharmacology. 2018;**84**(7):1432-1444

[34] Wang J, Leng SX. Inflammation and its role in ageing and disease. In: Oxford Textbook of Geriatric Medicine. Oxford University Press. Vol. 3. OUP Oxford; 2018

[35] American Geriatrics Society Beers Criteria® Update Expert Panel. American Geriatrics Society 2023 updated AGS Beers Criteria® for potentially inappropriate medication use in older adults. Journal of the American Geriatrics Society. 2023;**71**(7):2052-2081. DOI: 10.1111/jgs.18372

[36] Bahat G, Ilhan B, Erdogan T, Halil M, Savas S, Ulger Z, et al. Turkish inappropriate medication use in the elderly (TIME) criteria to improve prescribing in older adults: TIME-to-STOP/TIME-to-START. European Geriatric Medicine. 2020;**11**(3):491-498. DOI: 10.1007/s41999-020-00297-z

[37] Lavan AH, Gallagher P, Parsons C, O'Mahony D. STOPPFrail (screening tool of older persons' prescriptions in frail adults): Consensus validation. Age and Ageing. 2017;**46**(4):600-607. DOI: 10.1093/ageing/afx005

[38] Hanlon JT, Schmader KE, Samsa GP, Weinberger M, Uttech KM, Lewis IK, et al. A method for assessing drug therapy appropriateness. Journal of Clinical Epidemiology. 1992;**45**(10):1045-1051. DOI: 10.1016/0895-4356(92)90028-l

[39] Faniyi AA, Adnan MA, Tengku-Adnan TAS, Hashim NM, Tengku-Muhammad TS. Inflammation, ageing and diseases of the lung: Potential therapeutic strategies from shared biological pathways. British Journal of Pharmacology. 2022;**179**(9):1790-1807. DOI: 10.1111/bph.15804

[40] Morley JE, Vellas B, van Kan GA, Anker SD, Bauer JM, Bernabei R, et al. Frailty consensus: A call to action. Journal of the American Medical Directors Association. 2013;**14**(6):392-397. DOI: 10.1016/j.jamda.2013.03.022

[41] Cruz-Jentoft AJ, Bahat G, Bauer J, Boirie Y, Bruyère O, Cederholm T, et al. Sarcopenia: Revised European consensus on definition and diagnosis. Age and Ageing. 2019;**48**(1):16-31

[42] Cesari M, Nobili A, Vitale G. Frailty and sarcopenia: From theory to clinical implementation and public health relevance. European Journal of Internal Medicine. 2016;**35**:1-9

[43] Hoogendijk EO, Afilalo J, Ensrud KE, Kowal P, Onder G, Fried LP. Frailty: Implications for clinical practice and public health. Lancet. 2019;**394**(10206):1365-1375

[44] Hayes C, Yigezu A, Dillon S, Fitzgerald C, Manning M, Leahy A, et al. Home-based comprehensive geriatric assessment for community-dwelling, at-risk, frail older adults: A systematic review and meta-analysis. Journal of the American Geriatrics Society. 18 Feb 2025. DOI: 10.1111/jgs.19402 [Epub ahead of print]

[45] Chae HW, Kim Y, Suh Y, et al. Prevalence of potentially inappropriate

medications based on the STOPPFrail criteria in frail older patients with limited life expectancy: A cross-sectional study. BMC Geriatrics. 2022;**22**(1):367. DOI: 10.1186/s12877-022-03067-7

[46] Conlon M et al. Risk analysis index and its recalibrated version predict postoperative outcomes better than 5-factor modified frailty index in traumatic spinal injury. Neurospine. 2022;**19**(4):1039

[47] Chan WL et al. The predictive value of G8 and the Cancer and Aging Research Group chemotherapy toxicity tool in treatment-related toxicity in older Chinese patients with cancer. Journal of Geriatric Oncology. 2021;**12**(4):557-562

[48] Tumscitz C et al. Safety, efficacy and impact on frailty of mini-invasive radial balloon aortic valvuloplasty. Heart. 2021;**107**(11):874-880

[49] Kouroubali A et al. Developing an AI-enabled integrated care platform for frailty. Healthcare (Basel). 2022;**10**(3):443

[50] Orrall A. As lifespan increases, people spend more years burdened by disease. Journal of the American Medical Association. 2025;**333**(6):453. DOI: 10.1001/jama.2024.26884

[51] Fogg C, Fraser SDS, Roderick P, de Lusignan S, Clegg A, Brailsford S, et al. The dynamics of frailty development and progression in older adults in primary care in England (2006-2017): A retrospective cohort profile. BMJ Open. 2023;**13**(1):e063836. DOI: 10.1136/bmjopen-2022-063836

[52] Lorbergs AL, Prorok JC, Holroyd-Leduc J, et al. Nutrition and physical activity clinical practice guidelines for older adults living with frailty. The Journal of Frailty & Aging. 2022;**11**(1):3-11. DOI: 10.14283/jfa.2021.51

[53] Song S, Stern Y, Gu Y. Modifiable lifestyle factors and cognitive reserve: A systematic review of current evidence. Ageing Research Reviews. 2022;**74**:101551. DOI: 10.1016/j.arr.2021.101551

[54] Bian Z, Chen Y, Wu H, et al. Genetic predisposition, modifiable lifestyles, and their joint effects on human lifespan: Evidence from multiple cohort studies. BMJ Evidence-Based Medicine. 2024;**29**(4):255-263

[55] Dominguez LJ, Veronese N, Baiamonte R, et al. Rationale of the association between Mediterranean diet and the risk of frailty in older adults: A systematic review and meta-analysis. Experimental Gerontology. 2023;**177**:112180. DOI: 10.1016/j.exger.2023.112180

[56] Mulasso A, Rainero I, Roppolo M, et al. Effects of a multicomponent exercise program on prevalence and severity of the frailty syndrome in a sample of Italian community-dwelling older adults. Healthcare (Basel). 2022;**10**(5):807

[57] Bray NW, Smart RR, Jakobi JM. Multi-component exercise with high-intensity, free-weight, functional resistance training in pre-frail females: A quasi-experimental, pilot study. The Journal of Frailty & Aging. 2020;**9**(3):111-117

[58] Ye B, Zhang X, Liu M, et al. Psychological resilience and frailty progression in older adults. JAMA Network Open. 2024;7(11):e2447605. DOI: 10.1001/jamanetworkopen.2024.47605

[59] Kim ES, Kubzansky LD, VanderWeele TJ. Resilient aging:

Psychological well-being and social well-being as targets for the promotion of healthy aging. Journal of Gerontology & Geriatric Medicine. 2021;7:23337214211002951

[60] Jarach CM, Lugo A, Stival C, et al. Social isolation and loneliness as related to progression and reversion of frailty in the Survey of Health Aging Retirement in Europe (SHARE). Age and Ageing. 2021;**50**(1):258-262

[61] Yon Y, Mikton CR, Gassoumis ZD, Wilber KH. The prevalence of elder abuse in institutional settings: A systematic review and meta-analysis. European Journal of Public Health. 2019;**29**(1):58-67

[62] Beard JR, Officer A, de Carvalho IA, et al. The world report on ageing and health: A policy framework for healthy ageing. Lancet. 2016;**387**(10033):2145-2154

[63] Berkowitz RE, Fang Z, Helfand BK, et al. Project ReEngineered Discharge (RED) lowers hospital readmissions of patients discharged from a skilled nursing facility. Journal of the American Medical Directors Association. 2013;**14**(10):736-740. DOI: 10.1016/j.jamda.2013.03.003

[64] Fitzgerald KG, Caro FG. An overview of aging-friendly communities. American Journal of Preventive Medicine. 2014;**46**(3 Suppl. 1):S109-S114. DOI: 10.1016/j.amepre.2014.04.004

[65] World Health Organization. Decade of Healthy Ageing 2020-2030. Geneva: WHO; 2020. Available from: https://www.who.int/initiatives/decade-of-healthy-ageing [Accessed: May 6, 2025]

[66] Dent E, Morley JE, Cruz-Jentoft AJ, Woodhouse L, Rodríguez-Mañas L, Fried LP, et al. Physical frailty: ICFSR international clinical practice guidelines for identification and management. The Journal of Nutrition, Health & Aging. 2019;**23**(9):771-787. DOI: 10.1007/s12603-019-1273-z

[67] Li Y, Gao Y, Hu S, Chen H, Zhang M, Yang Y, et al. Effects of multicomponent exercise on the muscle strength, muscle endurance and balance of frail older adults: A meta-analysis of randomised controlled trials. Journal of Clinical Nursing. 2023;**32**(9-10):1795-1805. DOI: 10.1111/jocn.16196

[68] Rahi B, Ajana S, Tabue-Teguo M, Dartigues JF, Peres K, Féart C. High adherence to a Mediterranean diet and lower risk of frailty among French older adults community-dwellers: Results from the Three-City-Bordeaux study. Clinical Nutrition. 2018;**37**(4):1293-1298. DOI: 10.1016/j.clnu.2017.05.020

[69] Di Francesco A, Deighan AG, Litichevskiy L, et al. Dietary restriction impacts health and lifespan of genetically diverse mice. Nature. 2024;**634**:684-692. DOI: 10.1038/s41586-024-08026-3

[70] de Souza AF, de Oliveira DC, Ramírez PC, de Oliveira MR, Luiz MM, Delinocente MLB, et al. Low gait speed is better than frailty and sarcopenia at identifying the risk of disability in older adults. Age and Ageing. 2025;**54**(4):afaf104. DOI: 10.1093/ageing/afaf104

[71] Lim H, Jani NDB, Pang WT, Lim ECW. Community-based exercises improve health status in pre-frail older adults: A systematic review with meta-analysis. BMC Geriatrics. 2024;**24**(1):589. DOI: 10.1186/s12877-024-05150-7

[72] Racey M, Ali MU, Sherifali D, Fitzpatrick-Lewis D, Lewis R, Jovkovic M, et al. Effectiveness of physical activity interventions in older

adults with frailty or prefrailty: A systematic review and meta-analysis. CMAJ Open. 2021;**9**(3):E728-E743. DOI: 10.9778/cmajo.20200222

[73] Prestmo A, Hagen G, Sletvold O, Helbostad JL, Thingstad P, Taraldsen K, et al. Comprehensive geriatric care for patients with hip fractures: A prospective, randomised, controlled trial. Lancet. 2015;**385**(9978):1623-1633. DOI: 10.1016/S0140-6736(14)62409-0

[74] Oh S, Lee S. Effect of aquatic exercise on physical function and quality of life in individuals with neurological disorder: A systematic review and meta-analysis. Complementary Therapies in Clinical Practice. 2020;**39**:101164. DOI: 10.1016/j.ctcp.2020.101164

[75] Izquierdo M, Merchant RA, Morley JE, Anker SD, Aprahamian I, Arai H, et al. International exercise recommendations in older adults (ICFSR): Expert consensus guidelines. The Journal of Nutrition, Health & Aging. 2021;**25**(7):824-853. DOI: 10.1007/s12603-021-1665-8

[76] Tsolakidis D, Gymnopoulos LP, Dimitropoulos K. Artificial intelligence and machine learning technologies for personalized nutrition: A review. Informatics. 2024;**11**(3):62. DOI: 10.3390/informatics11030062

[77] Aliberti MJR, Bertola L, Szlejf C, Oliveira D, Piovezan RD, Cesari M, et al. Delivering patient-centered care: Outcomes of comprehensive geriatric assessment across healthcare settings. Geriatrics, Gerontology and Aging. 2022;**16**(4):e0220031. DOI: 10.5327/Z2447-211520222200031

Chapter 6

Beyond the Fracture: Mortality Risk and Survival after Hip Fractures in the Elderly

Eşref Selçuk

Abstract

Hip fractures in geriatric patients represent a critical public health challenge, leading to significant short- and long-term mortality and morbidity. As worldwide demographics shift toward an older age, the occurrence of hip fractures is expected to escalate sharply, placing increasing demands on healthcare systems. This manuscript reviews the biological underpinnings of aging, the epidemiology of hip fractures, early and late mortality risks, and the key role of frailty and multimorbidity in outcomes. Early surgical intervention, preferably within 24 to 48 hours, along with comprehensive perioperative and geriatric co-management strategies, is crucial for optimizing survival and recovery. Prognostic models can assist in risk stratification. Rehabilitation focusing on mobility, cognitive support, nutrition, and multidisciplinary collaboration is vital for restoring function and reducing secondary fractures. Despite advancements, there remains a need for standardized predictive tools and targeted interventions. Future research should prioritize patient-centered outcomes, early risk assessment, and real-world rehabilitation strategies to enhance quality of life and independence in this vulnerable population.

Keywords: hip fractures, mortality, geriatrics, risk factors, survival rate, frailty

1. Introduction

1.1 The global aging population

Across the world, populations are shifting dramatically as people live longer and birth rates decline. By 2050, the global population is expected to reach 9.7 billion, with over 2.1 billion individuals aged 60 and above. Notably, 80% of this population will reside in low- and middle-income countries [1]. The proportion of individuals aged 60 and older will nearly double from 12% in 2015 to 22% by 2050, while the number of those aged 80 and above is projected to triple, reaching 426 million.

These demographic changes create new challenges for health systems, elderly care, and social services. The rapid pace of population aging, particularly in resource-limited settings, necessitates integrated strategies that promote healthy aging, support chronic disease management, and ensure functional independence.

1.2 Biological foundations and heterogeneity of aging

Aging is a complex, multifactorial process characterized by progressive physiological decline. Hallmarks of biological aging include genomic instability, oxidative stress, telomere attrition, mitochondrial dysfunction, and cellular senescence [2]. These changes disrupt homeostasis and increase vulnerability to chronic disease.

Functional performance in older adults is closely linked to the combined effects of biological, behavioral, and social influences. Aging does not proceed in a uniform fashion; two individuals of the same age may exhibit markedly different levels of independence. Physical inactivity, poor nutrition, multiple medication use, and social isolation can speed up functional decline, while staying active, mentally engaged, and socially connected helps protect against it.

1.3 The clinical burden of age-related disease

Aging is strongly linked to a rise in noncommunicable diseases that significantly affect both physical and cognitive function. Common conditions among older adults include sensory impairments such as hearing loss and cataracts, which can limit communication and social engagement. Musculoskeletal disorders like osteoarthritis and osteoporosis cause chronic pain, decline in motor function, and increased tendency to fall [3].

Diseases like COPD make it harder to breathe and decrease how much exercise a person can handle. Metabolic disorders such as type 2 diabetes contribute to cardiovascular complications, neuropathy, and delayed wound healing. Neurodegenerative diseases, most notably Alzheimer's disease and dementia, gradually erode memory, cognition, and autonomy.

While each of these conditions has distinct pathophysiological mechanisms, they share a common underlying process: progressive molecular and cellular damage associated with aging [2]. Collectively, they increase vulnerability to falls, fractures, and long-term dependency while also prolonging recovery and complicating rehabilitation.

Among these complications, osteoporosis stands out as a major contributor to fracture risk, particularly hip fractures. Characterized by reduced bone mass and microarchitectural deterioration, osteoporosis greatly increases the likelihood of low-energy fractures in geriatric people. These fractures are especially serious, linked to substantial morbidity, diminished self-reliance, and high mortality. In 2019, the global incidence of hip fractures in individuals aged 55 and older was estimated at 681.35 per 100,000 population. One-year mortality following a hip fracture ranges between 2.4% and 34.8%, with an average of approximately 22%. These results highlight the major public health challenges that hip fractures create in geriatric populations [4].

1.4 Hip fracture

Hip fracture is a critical turning point in the health trajectory of older adults, often marking the shift from independent living to long-term disability. More than 90% of hip fractures take place in individuals aged 65 and over, usually after a low-energy fall [5]. This type of injury is not only a sign of underlying frailty but also a trigger for further health decline. Many patients lose mobility and are unable to regain baseline functional status.

Although the one-year mortality rate after a hip fracture ranges from 20 to 30%, this rate is comparable to the one-year mortality observed in several types of cancer. For example, early-stage cancers such as breast, thyroid, and prostate have a one-year mortality of approximately 1–3%, while colorectal and bladder cancers show rates of 5–10%. In contrast, more aggressive cancers like pancreatic, lung, and liver cancers can reach one-year mortality rates as high as 30–60% [6]. Beyond the immediate impact, hip fractures can start a downward spiral: prolonged immobility leads to muscle wasting, increased risk of complications like pneumonia or blood clots, and further cognitive or nutritional decline [7].

1.5 Comparative mortality: Hip fractures vs. other major diseases

When comparing the one-year mortality rates of hip fractures to other major health conditions, the seriousness becomes evident. For instance, the one-year mortality rate after an acute myocardial infarction in the elderly has declined during the past 15 years. Similarly, certain cancers have varying one-year mortality rates; for example, nonmetastatic breast cancer has a one-year mortality rate of approximately 1%, while metastatic cases can be significantly higher.

Notably, colorectal and stomach cancers exhibit one-year mortality rates that align closely with those observed in elderly patients following a hip fracture. According to the Surveillance, Epidemiology, and End Results (SEER) Program, colorectal cancer has a one-year mortality rate of approximately 20%, while stomach cancer's one-year mortality rate is around 30%.

These comparisons underscore that hip fractures can be as deadly, if not more so, than some forms of cancer or heart disease, emphasizing the need for preventive measures and effective management strategies.

2. Epidemiology

2.1 Global trends

Hip fractures represent a significant source of morbidity and mortality in the elderly population. Globally, the rate of hip fractures in people aged 55 years and above was reported to be 681.35 per 100,000 population in 2019, a figure that is projected to rise steadily with global population aging. By the year 2050, it is estimated that the annual number of hip fractures worldwide will reach approximately 6.26 million [5]. These projections underscore the growing burden of hip fractures on healthcare systems, particularly as the proportion of older adults continues to increase.

In a comprehensive review encompassing data over a 60-year period, Shahnawaz Haleem and colleagues observed a progressive increase in the mean age at which hip fractures occur, rising by approximately one year every five years [8]. In the 1960s, the average age at the time of hip fracture was 73 years, whereas by 2010, it had risen to 82 years. Interestingly, during the same period, 30-day mortality rates following hip fracture surgery showed a decline, dropping from 27 to 20%. This may reflect improvements in perioperative care, surgical techniques, and geriatric co-management strategies over the past several decades.

2.2 Age and gender differences

The hazard of hip fracture varies significantly by age and gender. In general, women are at higher risk than men, a disparity that becomes more pronounced after the age of 65. The decline in estrogen levels following menopause leads to reduced bone mineral density and a greater susceptibility to osteoporosis, thereby increasing fracture risk in female. In males, risk of fracture tends to rise at a later age. However, men exhibit higher mortality rates following hip fractures compared to women. This difference may be attributed to a higher prevalence of comorbid conditions and more severe postfracture complications in older men.

3. Early mortality after hip fracture

3.1 30-day and 90-day mortality

The first 90 days following a hip fracture represent a critical period during which the majority of fracture-related deaths occur. Numerous large-scale studies across various populations have consistently demonstrated that early mortality, particularly within the first month and quarter after injury, is substantial and deserves special attention in both clinical care and healthcare policy.

In a comprehensive nationwide study conducted in Sweden between 1998 and 2017, Nordström et al. reported an increase in one month mortality from 4.3% to 6.2% in female patients and from 8.4% to 11.1% among male patients over the study period, underscoring the persisting challenge of reducing early deaths after hip fracture despite advances in treatment and care.

Among institutionalized elderly individuals, Kilian Rapp and colleagues analyzed a cohort of newly admitted nursing home residents in Germany and found that 30-day mortality following a hip fracture was 16.1% in men and 10.1% in women. By comparison, age-, sex-, and care-level–matched controls without hip fracture had significantly lower mortality rates of 7.8% in men and 5.3% in women. Thus, hip fracture was linked to an absolute increase in 30-day mortality of 8.3% in men and 4.8% in women, corresponding to relative increases of 104.4% and 90.6%, respectively. At 90 days, mortality reached 34.1% in men and 22.8% in women with a hip fracture, compared to 17.9% and 14.0% in the control group, further emphasizing the disproportionate early mortality burden in male patients.

A recent systematic review and meta-analysis by Michael Bui et al. synthesizing data from over 460,000 patients has identified a median 30-day mortality rate of 8.0%. This benchmark aligns with data from individual institutional studies. For instance, Blanco et al. reported a 30-day mortality rate of 6.0% in a prospectively followed group of 923 people treated surgically. Similarly, in a Spanish matched cohort study by Gutiérrez-Misis and colleagues, the 30-day mortality rate among elderly patients with hip fracture was 6.1%, compared to just 0.3% in community-dwelling individuals without fracture. The hip fracture elevates the risk of death within 30 days by a factor of 8.4 (HR: 8.4, $p < 0.001$).

In our own retrospective cohort study conducted at Trakya University, we analyzed data from 356 people with ages of 82.9 ± 8.3 years. The 30-day mortality rate was found to be 12.7%, while the 90-day mortality rate reached 32.7%. Notably, 70.1% of all deaths occurring within the first year took place during the initial 90 days, reinforcing the concept that the early postoperative phase is the most vulnerable period for this patient population.

Shen et al. investigated early outcomes in 1096 patients aged 70 and older who underwent hip arthroplasty during the COVID-19 pandemic. Their multicenter retrospective study reported a 90-day mortality rate of 5.2%. Although lower than in some earlier studies, these reflect a carefully selected surgical population during a period of heightened clinical vigilance.

Finally, a large Canadian study by Beaupre and colleagues involving 11,996 patients reported 30- and 90-day mortality rates of 4.9% and 8.5%, respectively. These results further contribute to the body of evidence confirming that hip fracture in geriatric linked to early mortality, which peaks within the first 3 months post-injury.

Based on the available data, 30-day mortality following hip fracture ranges from a minimum of 4.3% (among female patients in the Swedish nationwide study) to a maximum of 16.1% (among male nursing home residents in the study).

Collectively, these results highlight the need for aggressive perioperative optimization, early mobilization, and targeted multidisciplinary management strategies to reduce early mortality following hip fractures, particularly in vulnerable subgroups such as the very elderly, institutionalized individuals, and men.

3.2 Risk factors for early death

Early mortality following hip fracture surgery is most commonly classified as death occurring within one month postoperatively. In a comprehensive systematic review and meta-analysis conducted by Michael Bui and colleagues, five preoperative risk factors were consistently associated with significantly increased 30-day mortality: advanced age (OR: 1.06 per year), ASA score ≥ 3 (OR: 2.69), male sex (OR: 2.00), institutional residence (OR: 1.81), and presence of metastatic cancer (OR: 2.83). These variables have been repeatedly validated as critical determinants in early postoperative outcomes.

A prospective cohort study by Blanco et al. involving patients over the age of 65 who underwent hip fracture surgery further highlighted several independent predictors of 30-day mortality. Among them, chronic heart failure emerged as the strongest factor (OR: 3.560; $p < 0.001$), followed by elevated ASA classification (≥3) (OR: 3.273; $p < 0.001$) and use of oral anticoagulants (OR: 2.499; $p = 0.002$). Hypoalbuminemia (serum albumin ≤3.5 g/dL) (OR: 2.474) and arrhythmia (OR: 2.523) were also significantly linked to increased early mortality risk.

In a matched-cohort study conducted in Spain, key predictors of 30-day mortality included advanced age, high comorbidity burden as measured by a Charlson Comorbidity Index ≥3 (HR: 2.59), and functional disability (defined as dependence in ≥2 basic activities of daily living; HR: 1.22). Interestingly, cognitive impairment was not significantly associated with mortality at 30 days, though it became a relevant factor at 3 and 12 months. Although male sex appeared to be linked to short-term mortality in univariate analysis, its significance did not persist in multivariate models.

In our own retrospective study conducted at Trakya University, advanced age was found to be a statistically significant predictor of 30-day mortality (OR: 1.11) with each additional year of age increasing the risk. Male sex also emerged as an independent risk factor (OR: 1.87), with men demonstrating a higher mortality risk than women. Additional predictors of early mortality included the need for postoperative intensive care (OR: 2.14) and prolonged hospitalization (OR: 1.03). Furthermore, comorbid conditions such as malignancy (OR: 3.44), cerebrovascular disease (OR: 2.07), and chronic respiratory disorders (OR: 3.49) were also strongly associated with early postoperative death.

Shen et al., in a multicenter retrospective analysis, examined 1096 elderly patients undergoing hip arthroplasty and identified four key preoperative risk factors for 90-day mortality through multivariate logistic regression: chronic obstructive pulmonary disease (OR: 2.10), dementia (OR: 3.00), and prolonged time from fracture to surgery (OR: 1.11). Their findings underscore the critical need to address both medical and procedural delays in surgical planning.

Finally, in a large cohort study of 11,996 patients, Beaupre and colleagues confirmed that advanced age (≥85 years), male sex, elevated Charlson Comorbidity Index (≥2), and surgical delay were all independently associated with 90-day mortality. Notably, older patients were found to be more susceptible to the adverse effects of delayed surgery, with mortality risk increasing with each hour of delay.

These findings from these diverse studies conducted across multiple healthcare systems highlight several consistent preoperative risk factors for early (30- to 90-day) mortality following operation. Advanced age, male sex, high comorbidity burden (often quantified by a Charlson Comorbidity Index ≥2 or 3), and elevated ASA scores (≥3) emerge as the most frequently reported and robust predictors. Additionally, clinical indicators such as hypoalbuminemia, chronic heart failure, arrhythmia, malignancy, and chronic respiratory disease are recurrently linked to poorer outcomes. Delays in surgical intervention also appear to significantly worsen early prognosis, particularly in the oldest patient groups. These findings underscore the importance of a timely, comprehensive preoperative evaluation that integrates both functional and clinical risk profiles. Optimizing modifiable risk factors and prioritizing early surgical management, especially in high-risk patients, may offer a valuable opportunity to reduce early mortality rates following hip fractures.

4. Long-term survival and prognosis

4.1 1-year and 5-year survival

Recent studies have highlighted both improvements and ongoing challenges in hip fracture outcomes. Shahnawaz Haleem and colleagues, analyzing data over the past six decades, stated that the one year mortality rate decreased from 27% in the 1960s to 20% in the 2010s, reflecting advances in prevention, medical care, specialized orthogeriatric units, and timely surgery [8]. In Taiwan, Kun-Han Lee et al. highlighted that 1-year mortality rates were 23.3% for collum femoris fracture and 26.6% trochanteric fractures, while 10-year mortality outcomes were notably higher, at 69.3% and 74.3%, respectively [9, 10]. Similarly, a Spanish study by Olalla Guzon-Illescas et al. involving 3992 patients showed a 1-year mortality rate of 33%, with higher rates observed in men (43.3%) compared to women (30%) [10].

In a population-based register study from Denmark by Michael Houlind Larsen et al., using data from the Danish National Patient Registry between 1998 and 2017, the 1-year (365-day) mortality rate after surgically treated femoral fractures in patients aged 65 and older was 29% overall, with 37% in men and 26% in women [11]. Also, the study demonstrated that high mortality rates are not limited to proximal femoral fractures but extend across all femoral fracture locations, including diaphyseal and distal femur fractures.

In a retrospective single-center study conducted in China by Pingping Wang and Shenghua Guo, elderly patients with femoral neck fractures who underwent joint replacement surgery were evaluated to determine the impact of multiple chronic conditions (MCC) on postoperative mortality [12]. The study revealed that patients with MCC experienced significantly higher mortality rates compared to those without. Specifically, 1-year mortality outcomes among people with MCC were 28.2% (29 out of 103), while the 5-year mortality rate reached 40.8% (42 out of 103). These findings underscore the prognostic importance of comorbidity burden in elderly patients undergoing surgical treatment for femoral neck fractures.

In an analysis of past clinical data, 766 elderly people who underwent surgical treatment for hip fractures between 2007 and 2009 were monitored for at least 10 years to identify predictors for long-term mortality [13]. The study reported a one-year mortality of 12.0%, a 5-year mortality rate of 38.9%, and a 10-year mortality rate of 61.6%.

Through a review of cohort from Japan by Kenji Shigemoto et al., 678 geriatric people with proximal femur fractures were treated using a multidisciplinary care model at Toyama City Hospital between 2014 and 2018 [14]. The 1-year mortality rate was reported as 12.6%, with elevated mortality in males (20.7%) compared to females (10.5%).

In a retrospective single-center study conducted in Turkey by Olgun Bingöl et al., the 1-year mortality outcome among 241 geriatric people with hip fractures was stated as 25.3% [15].

In a retrospective cohort study conducted in Türkiye, 346 geriatric patients who operated for hip fractures at Trakya University were analyzed to evaluate the COVID-19 on mortality outcomes [16]. This study found 1-year mortality rate of 49.1% in the pre-COVID era and 43.9% during the COVID era, with an overall 1-year mortality outcome of 46.5%. The findings highlight the persistently high mortality with geriatric hip fractures.

4.2 Predictors of long-term outcomes

Hip fractures in the geriatric patients are linked to high mortality rates extending well beyond the immediate postoperative period. Numerous studies have sought to identify reliable predictors of one-year and longer-term mortality to guide perioperative care and improve outcomes in this vulnerable population [11, 13].

Advanced age consistently emerges as a strong independent predictor of mortality. Incremental increases in age are associated with proportionally higher risk of death, with some studies reporting hazard ratios exceeding 1.10 per year. Male sex is also associated with poorer survival, with men exhibiting significantly higher mortality rates than women across multiple national datasets.

Comorbidity burden is another well-established determinant of long-term survival [9, 10, 12]. Quantitative indices such as the Charlson Comorbidity Index (CCI) and age-adjusted CCI (ACCI) demonstrate a clear correlation with mortality. Patients with multiple chronic conditions or higher ACCI scores show markedly reduced survival, with 10-year mortality rates exceeding 70% in high-risk groups. In addition to aggregate indices, specific comorbidities such as chronic pulmonary disease, cerebrovascular disease, renal insufficiency, and malignancy have been independently associated with worse outcomes.

Recent evidence has also highlighted the prognostic value of inflammatory markers. Elevated neutrophil-to-lymphocyte ratio (NLR) and monocyte-to-lymphocyte ratio (MLR) at admission have been linked to increased mortality risk at both 30 days and one year [15]. These markers may reflect underlying systemic inflammation and frailty and provide an accessible means of early risk stratification.

Timing of surgery plays a critical role in survival. Delays in operative intervention beyond 48 hours are associated with a significant increase in one-year mortality, with some studies estimating a 10–15% rise in risk for each additional day [16, 17]. This association underscores the importance of expedited surgical care in reducing adverse outcomes.

Postoperative intensive care unit (ICU) admission has also been associated with increased mortality, suggesting that patients requiring ICU care represent a particularly vulnerable subset. Limited physiological reserve, higher perioperative complication rates, and delayed mobilization may contribute to this finding.

In conclusion, mortality over time is influenced by age, sex, comorbidities, inflammatory status, surgical timing, and postoperative course. Identification of these predictors enables early risk stratification and may inform targeted interventions to reduce mortality and enhance recovery in older adults undergoing hip fracture surgery.

5. Frailty and comorbidities

5.1 Frailty indexes and tools

Frailty is increasingly recognized as a critical factor influencing outcomes in elderly patients, particularly those undergoing orthopedic procedures such as hip fracture surgery. It reflects a decline across multiple physiological systems, resulting in reduced resilience to medical and surgical stressors [18]. Frail individuals have a greater chance of experiencing complications, longer hospital stays, institutionalization, functional decline, and mortality, even when receiving standard-of-care treatment.

Two primary conceptual models are used to assess frailty [7, 19]. The Fried physical phenotype identifies frailty with 5 observable indicators: involuntary weight decrease, fatigue, reduced strength, reduced gait speed, and reduced activity level. This model classifies patients as robust, pre-frail, or frail, depending on how many criteria they meet. Alternatively, the Cumulative Deficit Model, developed by Rockwood and colleagues, views frailty as the accumulation of health deficits, including comorbidities, symptoms, and functional impairments, and expresses it as a Frailty Index (FI). This index enables a graded assessment of frailty severity, which is especially useful for risk stratification in heterogeneous elderly populations.

Beyond these models, more comprehensive tools have been developed to reflect the multidimensional nature of frailty. One of the most robust and clinically applicable is the Multidimensional Prognostic Index (MPI), obtained from Comprehensive Geriatric Assessment (CGA). The MPI contained eight domains: mobility, mental performance, comorbidities, nutritional status, multiple medication, risk of pressure ulcers, social support, and cohabitation status. Patients are classified into three categories—robust (MPI < 0.33), pre-frail (0.34–0.66), and frail (>0.66)—each with clearly defined prognostic implications.

Meta-analyses have demonstrated that MPI-defined frailty is highly prevalent, particularly in nursing homes (>50%) and hospitals (~30%) [20, 21]. Crucially, high MPI scores are independently linked to greater frequency of surgical complications, institutionalization, and one-year mortality in geriatric orthopedic patients. Preoperative frailty, regardless of how it is measured, has been shown to significantly predict poor postoperative recovery and survival.

In this context, frailty assessment is more than a prognostic exercise; it serves as a clinical decision-making tool. In elderly patients who are socially isolated, cognitively impaired, or burdened by multiple comorbidities, structured frailty evaluations such as the MPI can guide the choice of surgical versus conservative treatment, help anticipate perioperative needs, and support discharge planning. Furthermore, frailty screening aligns with ethical and patient-centered care principles, helping clinicians balance risks and benefits while aligning medical interventions with the patient's goals and values.

Given the rising prevalence of frailty in aging societies and the growing orthopedic burden it entails, integrating frailty screening into routine preoperative assessment is not only justified, it is imperative.

5.2 Multiple chronic conditions

Multimorbidity, representing the coexistence of several persistent illnesses, is highly prevalent among older adults with hip fractures and exerts a substantial influence on both short- and long-term outcomes. The presence of multiple comorbidities complicates perioperative management and contributes to an elevated risk of complications, functional decline, and mortality.

In a nationwide Danish registry-based study involving over 92,000 patients, Hansen et al. demonstrated a strong interaction between multimorbidity and the risk of postoperative infections following hip fracture surgery [22]. Patients with high comorbidity burden (Charlson Comorbidity Index $\geq$3) exhibited a one-month infection rate of 302 per 100 person-years, in contrast to only 9 per 100 person-years among patients without multimorbidity. Notably, 33% of infections in the severely multimorbid group were directly attributable to the combined effect of hip fracture surgery and multimorbidity.

Beyond the acute setting, multimorbidity also affects long-term outcomes. In a 12-year European prospective cohort study, Veronese et al. observed that older adults with multimorbidity who engaged in regular physical activity had up to 51% lower all-cause mortality compared to sedentary individuals [23]. These findings suggest that physical activity may serve as a protective factor capable of mitigating some of the excess mortality associated with multimorbidity in hip fracture patients.

In terms of secondary prevention, a Canadian population-based cohort study by Ali et al. revealed a paradoxical pattern in osteoporosis care delivery [24]. While patients with two comorbidities were more likely to receive osteoporosis treatment following a fragility fracture, those with three or more comorbid conditions were significantly less likely to initiate therapy. This indicates a care gap potentially driven by therapeutic inertia in patients perceived as too frail or complex for standard treatment regimens.

Collectively, these findings underscore the multifaceted impact of multimorbidity in the context of geriatric hip fracture care. Not only does it increase biological vulnerability, but it also influences infection risk, survival probability, and the likelihood of receiving evidence-based interventions. Addressing these challenges requires a multidisciplinary approach that integrates orthopedic, geriatric, and rehabilitative expertise and prioritizes individualized, goal-directed care planning for this high-risk population.

6. Timing of surgery and perioperative management

6.1 Early vs. delayed surgery

Timely surgical intervention following hip fracture is widely regarded as a cornerstone of effective management in elderly patients. Clinical guidelines, including those from the American Academy of Orthopedic Surgeons, suggest operation in 48 hours from time of patient intake to reduce risk of complications and mortality [25]. Several high-quality studies reinforce the clinical value of early surgery compared to delayed intervention.

Shen et al. conducted a retrospective analysis in a Taiwanese medical center, including 1118 geriatric patients with hip fractures [26]. The authors demonstrated that waiting more than 36 hours for surgery significantly increased the incidence of pneumonia (4.4% vs. 7.9%), myocardial infarction (3.0% vs. 7.2%), and heart failure (15.2% vs. 26.8%) within the first 30 days postoperatively. These complications persisted at 90 days, highlighting the time-sensitive nature of surgical care.

Lieten et al. analyzed over 800 cases in Belgium and found that patients undergoing surgery within 24 hours had significantly lower rates of cardiovascular and pulmonary complications [27]. Delayed surgery (mean time to surgery: 73 hours) was linked to worse long-term outcomes (OR: 2.63, $p < 0.001$). A delayed surgery was associated with a twofold increase in mortality. And survival analysis showed that early surgical intervention significantly improved survival outcomes.

Bhatti et al. utilized the National Trauma Data Bank (NTDB) in the United States, encompassing 28,031 elderly patients [28]. The authors found that patients receiving surgery within 48 hours had a mortality rate of 1.6%, compared to 4.2% in the delayed group ($p < 0.001$). Sociodemographic disparities such as race, hospital region, and injury severity were also associated with delays, indicating potential systemic factors influencing timeliness of care.

Joseph et al. provided a nuanced perspective by demonstrating that delays beyond 48 hours were associated with increased cardiology consultations and a higher comorbidity burden. However, the 1-year mortality was similar between the early and delayed surgery groups in their cohort ($p = 0.109$) [29]. However, a Cox proportional hazards model indicated a small but statistically significant increase in mortality risk with each hour of delay (HR: 1.007; $p = 0.001$), suggesting that even minor surgical delays may have cumulative effects.

Collectively, these studies confirm that early surgical intervention, preferably within 24 to 48 hours, is linked to low rates of cardiopulmonary complications and improved survival result in geriatric patients with hip fractures. While individual patient optimization remains important, unnecessary surgical delays, particularly due to logistical or administrative factors, may result in avoidable harm. A system-wide commitment to prioritizing early surgery can significantly impact outcomes in this vulnerable population.

6.2 Anesthesia considerations

Types of anesthesia in geriatric patients undergoing hip fracture operations greatly impact operative results, particularly given the high prevalence of frailty, multimorbidity, and cognitive impairment in this population. The most commonly used techniques are general anesthesia and spinal anesthesia, each with specific advantages and limitations. Additionally, regional nerve blocks and emerging local anesthesia protocols such as MAC-STILA (Monitored Anesthesia Care with Soft

Tissue Infiltration of Local Anesthetics) are gaining interest for their potential to reduce complications in high-risk patients.

General vs. Spinal Anesthesia

General anesthesia provides reliable analgesia and is often necessary for complex cases but is associated with risks such as hemodynamic instability, postoperative delirium, and respiratory complications. Spinal anesthesia offers hemodynamic benefits and eliminates the need for airway instrumentation, and several studies have associated it with lower rates of early complications, though recent randomized trials such as the REGAIN trial have found no significant difference in 60-day functional outcomes or mortality between general and spinal anesthesia [30].

Peripheral Nerve Blocks and Multimodal Analgesia

Contemporary guidelines emphasize the use of regional nerve blocks (e.g., femoral, fascia iliaca, PENG block) both as standalone techniques and adjuncts to general or spinal anesthesia. These blocks improve preoperative pain control, reduce opioid requirements, and may decrease rate of postoperative delirium encourage early mobilization [30, 31].

Novel Local Anesthesia Techniques: MAC-STILA

Emerging evidence supports the role of MAC-STILA as an alternative in medically fragile patients. This technique combines light intravenous sedation with targeted local anesthetic infiltration at key surgical sites. Pilot studies suggest that MAC-STILA results in improved intraoperative physiological stability, lower postoperative pain and delirium rates, and comparable outcomes to spinal and general anesthesia without the need for airway manipulation [32].

6.3 Geriatric co-management

Orthogeriatric co-management is a multidisciplinary care model that integrates orthopedic surgeons and geriatricians in the joint management of older adults with hip fractures across both acute and rehabilitation phases. The rationale stems from the recognition that elderly patients with fragility fractures often suffer from multimorbidity, frailty, cognitive impairment, and functional decline, factors that increase the risk of poor outcomes if managed in a surgery-only framework.

Yee et al. demonstrated that implementing an orthogeriatric collaboration pathway led to improved patient outcomes [33]. In this model, shared ward rounds were conducted, patients were transferred to rehabilitation more quickly, and continuous geriatric oversight was provided. As a result, the length of stay was reduced in both acute hospitals (median 7 vs. 8 days) and rehabilitation centers (16 vs. 18 days). Patients also showed better functional recovery at discharge, measured by the Modified Barthel Index, and there was a higher rate of osteoporosis treatment initiation. Importantly, these improvements were achieved without increasing mortality or hospital readmission rates.

De Vincentis et al. emphasized through a nationwide Italian consensus that effective co-management requires a multidisciplinary team (MDT) composed of at least an orthopedic surgeon, anesthesiologist, and geriatrician, supported by physiatrists and physiotherapists [34]. The consensus outlines evidence-based recommendations covering:

- Preoperative optimization (e.g., comprehensive geriatric assessment),
- Perioperative management (e.g., early surgery, delirium prevention),

- Postoperative rehabilitation,
- Discharge planning and caregiver involvement.
- Both sources converge on the conclusion that orthogeriatric co-management is associated with improved clinical outcomes, greater system efficiency, and more personalized, function-oriented care for a growing elderly population.

7. Prognostic models and scoring systems

7.1 Nottingham hip fracture score

The Nottingham Hip Fracture Score (NHFS) is a validated preoperative hazard stratification system developed to estimate the 30-day mortality risk in geriatric patients. First introduced in 2007, the NHFS integrates seven objective clinical variables routinely available at hospital admission: Age, Sex, Hemoglobin level, Mini-Mental Test Score, Presence ≥2 comorbidities, Diagnosis of malignancy, Pre-admission residence (institutionalized vs. home).

Each variable contributes a defined number of points, and the total score (ranging from 0 to 10) corresponds to an estimated mortality percentage. For example, a score of 0 corresponds to < 1% mortality, while a score of 10 reflects ~ 45% 30-day mortality risk [35].

Recent studies have shown that the NHFS also has moderate predictive value for 1-year mortality and can aid in guiding perioperative decisions, family discussions, and resource planning [36]. When compared with the Clinical Frailty Scale (CFS), NHFS has slightly better discrimination in predicting mortality, although both tools are complementary.

The NHFS is practical, bedside-applicable, and does not rely on intraoperative variables, making it particularly valuable for early triage and counseling in emergency orthopedic settings.

7.2 Charlson comorbidity index

The Charlson Comorbidity Index (CCI) is commonly employed clinical tool designed to quantify the burden of comorbid diseases and estimate a patient's 1-year mortality risk. The index assigns weighted scores to 19 chronic conditions (e.g., heart failure, diabetes, and cancer), with additional points for age, creating an Age-adjusted CCI (ACCI) commonly used in geriatric populations.

Recent findings have extended the application of CCI beyond mortality prediction. A 2022 study by Wong et al. demonstrated that a higher ACCI score is significantly associated with early fracture-related complications in elderly patients undergoing internal fixation for femoral neck fractures [37].

8. Preventive strategies and rehabilitation

8.1 Secondary prevention

Secondary prevention refers to healthcare services aimed at identifying a disease at an early stage and preventing its progression and complications. In short, the goal is not to completely prevent the disease, but to intervene early to stop it from worsening. For example, in orthopedics, systems such as Fracture Liaison Services have been developed. These focus on initiating appropriate and adequate treatment for osteoporosis following a fracture, ensuring that osteoporosis management is started in a timely manner.

Another cost-effective program microsimulation model for secondary fracture prevention was developed by Nayak et al. [38]. This model would prevented approximately 30,000 fractures per 1 million patients over 5 years, with a cost savings of $418 per patient.

Effective secondary prevention involves systematic identification of patients, bone mineral density measurement, appropriate anti-osteoporotic treatment (bisphosphonates, RANKL inhibitor, teriparatide, and sclerastin inhibitor), and multidisciplinary follow-up.

Additionally, secondary prevention efforts are more cost-effective when targeted to high-risk groups, such as institutionalized elderly individuals, and when using low-cost treatments like calcium plus vitamin D or hormonal therapy, as supported by long-term economic analyses.

8.2 Fall prevention programs

Falls are the leading cause of hip fractures among older adults; thus, structured fall prevention programs are essential in reducing fracture incidence. The multifactorial nature of fall risk—encompassing sarcopenia, visual impairment, polypharmacy, balance deficits, and environmental hazards—necessitates a comprehensive, individualized approach.

According to a 2023 review by Yu et al., recent evidence has highlighted several modifiable fall-related risk factors [39]:

- Neuromuscular impairment,
- Visual dysfunction,
- Use of psychotropic or antihypertensive medications,
- Malnutrition and electrolyte disorders (e.g., hyponatremia),
- Sedation due to opioid or analgesic overuse.
- Recommended strategies include:
- Exercise programs focusing on balance, strength, and gait training.
- Medication review and deprescribing, particularly of high-risk drugs like benzodiazepines or opioids.
- Environmental modifications, especially in home settings (e.g., removing loose rugs, improving lighting).
- Use of external hip protectors, which have been shown to reduce impact in case of falls.
- Vitamin D supplementation, at doses of 800–1000 IU daily, which has been associated with fall and fracture risk reduction.

When implemented within coordinated geriatric care frameworks, these programs not only improve quality of life but also reduce healthcare utilization and long-term disability. Geriatric rehabilitation following hip fracture is a cornerstone of recovery, aiming to reduce mortality, restore function, and prevent subsequent fractures. These programs rely on a multidisciplinary approach, early mobilization, individualized goal-setting, and seamless care transitions.

8.3 Rehabilitation

The main goals of geriatric rehabilitation programs are to help patients regain as much of their pre-fracture functional status as possible [40]. Restoring independence in daily activities is a key focus. It is also important to prevent complications such as malnutrition, delirium, and immobility syndrome, which are common with prolonged inactivity. Rehabilitation aims to reduce the need for long-term institutional care and maintain the patient's quality of life. In addition, targeted interventions are used to decline the hazard of secondary fractures by addressing osteoporosis and fall prevention.

8.3.1 Multidisciplinary team

Effective rehabilitation requires a coordinated team involving geriatricians, physiotherapists, occupational therapists, nurses, dietitians, social workers, and psychologists. Each member contributes to a personalized care plan tailored to the patient's physical, cognitive, and social needs [41, 42].

8.3.2 Early initiation of rehabilitation

Evidence-based guidelines recommend that rehabilitation begin within 6 days postoperatively. Early intervention is associated with better functional outcomes and reduced mortality [42, 43].

8.3.3 Functional and mobility training

Progressive weight-bearing, gait training, balance exercises, and resistance therapy are the mainstays. Therapy intensity typically ranges from 120 to 180 minutes daily [44]. Activities of daily living are integrated as therapeutic opportunities.

8.3.4 Cognitive and psychosocial support

Given the high prevalence of delirium, depression, and dementia in this population, cognitive screening and psychological support are integral. Patient and caregiver education is also emphasized.

8.3.5 Nutritional and comorbidity management

Due to the high risk of malnutrition, tailored dietary interventions by registered dietitians are essential [45]. Concurrently, medical management of heart failure, urinary infections, thromboembolism, and osteoporosis is necessary to prevent setbacks.

8.3.6 Barriers and enablers

In a qualitative study by Backman et al., the most significant barriers to early rehabilitation access included limited bed availability, inadequate staffing, and care coordination challenges [42]. Key enablers were effective patients and family counseling, consciousness of rehabilitation gains, and training in standardized care pathways.

8.3.7 Predicting duration and optimizing planning

A 2024 study by Krakers et al. identified several predictors of rehabilitation length of stay in skilled nursing facilities: post-discharge mobility level (Functional Ambulation Categories), surgery type, weight-bearing restrictions, presence of in-hospital delirium or heart failure, and pre-fracture living situation [46]. Anticipating these factors can support realistic goal-setting and efficient resource allocation.

9. Future research

Despite advancements in both surgical techniques and rehabilitation, many aspects in the care of elderly patients remain to be clarified. First, standardized predictive models should integrate frailty, comorbidity indices, and inflammatory markers. There is a need for multicenter, long-term data supported by early surgical intervention and co-management models. Given the variability in rehabilitation resources across different healthcare systems and socioeconomic settings, future efforts should focus on identifying optimal rehabilitation strategies. Bridging these gaps will be critical in improving long-term outcomes.

Future research should be prospective, multicenter, and randomized controlled. These studies should incorporate frailty indices, novel biomarkers, and comorbidity scores. New composite prognostic models need to be developed, aligned with real-world settings. They should focus on patient-centered outcomes, including the ability to live independently and overall quality of life, and also aim to identify and address caregiver burden.

10. Conclusion

Geriatric hip fractures are a significant orthopedic public health issue. They are associated with high mortality in both the early and late periods. Early surgical intervention, a multidisciplinary approach, and geriatric rehabilitation are essential. Frailty and multimorbidity remain among the most critical challenges during treatment and rehabilitation. Despite advancements, future research should focus on developing standardized, patient-centered models to improve survival, function, and quality of life in this growing population.

Conflict of interest

The authors declare no conflict of interest.

Appendices and nomenclature

AAOS	American academy of orthopedic surgeons
ACCI	age-adjusted Charlson comorbidity index
ASA	American society of anesthesiologists (score)
CCI	Charlson comorbidity index
CGA	comprehensive geriatric assessment
COPD	chronic obstructive pulmonary disease
FI	frailty index
HR	hazard ratio
MAC-STILA	monitored anesthesia care with soft tissue infiltration of local anesthetics
MCC	multiple chronic conditions
MPI	multidimensional prognostic index
MDT	multidisciplinary team
NHFS	Nottingham hip fracture score
NLR	neutrophil-to-lymphocyte ratio
OR	odds ratio
SEER	surveillance, epidemiology, and end results program
Hip Fracture	A break occurring in the proximal femur.
Frailty	A multidimensional syndrome characterized by decreased physiological reserve and resistance to stressors, leading to increased vulnerability to adverse health outcomes.
Multimorbidity	The coexistence of two or more chronic health conditions in an individual, often complicating treatment and prognosis.
Secondary Prevention	Medical interventions aimed at detecting and treating a disease early to halt its progression and prevent complications.
Early Mortality	Death occurring within 30 to 90 days after an index event (e.g., surgery for hip fracture).
Geriatric Co-Management	An interdisciplinary care approach where orthopedic surgeons and geriatricians jointly manage elderly patients to optimize perioperative outcomes and rehabilitation.
Functional Recovery	The process by which a patient regains physical, cognitive, and social abilities after an injury or illness to approach their baseline functional status.

Author details

Eşref Selçuk
Department of Orthopedics and Traumatology, Trakya University Faculty of Medicine, Edirne, Turkey

*Address all correspondence to: trkesref@hotmail.com

References

[1] World Health Organization. Decade of Healthy Ageing: Baseline Report. Geneva: World Health Organization; 2020

[2] López-Otín C, Blasco MA, Partridge L, Serrano M, Kroemer G. The hallmarks of aging. Cell. 2013;**153**:1194-1217

[3] Noto S. Perspectives on aging and quality of life. Healthcare (Switzerland). 2023;**11**:2131, 1-11. DOI: 10.3390/healthcare11152131

[4] Nan FJ, Gui ZC, Hua LB, Yan ZS, Feng WS, Li SC. Global burden of hip fracture: The global burden of disease study. Osteoporosis International. 2024;**35**(1):41-52. DOI: 10.1007/s00198-023-06907-3

[5] Schmid T, Brumme U, Kemerle S, Zimmer K. Elderly osteoporosis suspects without diagnosis—Interim data from a German geriatric practice. Value in Health. 2015;**18**:A654. DOI: 10.1016/j.jval.2015.09.2361

[6] Siegel RL, Miller KD, Wagle NS, Jemal A. Cancer statistics, 2023. CA: A Cancer Journal for Clinicians. 2023;**73**(1):17-48. DOI: 10.3322/caac.21763

[7] Fried LP, Tangen CM, Walston J, Newman AB, Hirsch C, Gottdiener J, et al. Frailty in older adults: Evidence for a phenotype. Journals of Gerontology - Series A Biological Sciences and Medical Sciences. 2001;**56**(3):M146-M156. DOI: 10.1093/gerona/56.3.m146

[8] Haleem S, Choudri MJ, Kainth GS, Parker MJ. Mortality following hip fracture: Trends and geographical variations over the last SIXTY years. Injury. 2023;**54**(2):620-629. DOI: 10.1016/j.injury.2022.12.008

[9] Lee K-H, Shih K-S, Hou S-M, Chen C-C, Peng T-Y, Liu Y-C, et al. Long-term survival outcome of patients with femoral neck and trochanteric fractures: A nationwide population-based observational study. Asian Journal of Surgery. 2025;**48**(5):2897-2901

[10] Guzon-Illescas O, Perez Fernandez E, Crespí Villarias N, Quirós Donate FJ, Peña M, Alonso-Blas C, et al. Mortality after osteoporotic hip fracture: Incidence, trends, and associated factors. Journal of Orthopaedic Surgery and Research. 2019;**14**(1):203. DOI: 10.1186/s13018-019-1226-6

[11] Larsen MH, Gundtoft PH, Viberg B. High mortality among elderly with surgical treated femoral fracture in comparison to other surgical treated lower extremity fractures: A population-based register study from the Danish National Patient Registry. Injury. 2025;**56**:112176, 1-7. DOI: 10.1016/j.injury.2025.112176

[12] Wang P, Guo S. Correlation between Charlson comorbidity index and surgical prognosis in elderly patients with femoral neck fractures: A retrospective study. BMC Musculoskeletal Disorders. 2024;**25**:678, 1-13. DOI: 10.1186/s12891-024-07814-2

[13] Loh B, Jiang L, Timing L, Kong N, Ganesan G, Tan KB, et al. Predictors of 10-year mortality after hip fracture surgery in a pre-pandemic cohort. Geriatric Orthopaedic Surgery and Rehabilitation. 2023;**14**:1-6. DOI: 10.1177/21514593231216558

[14] Shigemoto K, Sawaguchi T, Horii T, Goshima K, Iwai S, Higashikawa T, et al. Multidisciplinary care model for geriatric patients with hip fracture in Japan: 5-year

experience. Archives of Orthopaedic and Trauma Surgery. 2022;**142**(9):2205-2214. DOI: 10.1007/s00402-021-03933-w

[15] Bingol O, Ozdemir G, Kulakoglu B, Keskin OH, Korkmaz I, Kilic E. Admission neutrophil-to-lymphocyte ratio and monocyte-to-lymphocyte ratio to predict 30-day and 1-year mortality in geriatric hip fractures. Injury. 2020;**51**(11):2663-2667. DOI: 10.1016/j.injury.2020.07.048

[16] Eşref S, Murat E, Gökçen SE, Oğuz M. The impact of the COVID-19 pandemic on one-year mortality in geriatric hip fracture: A retrospective cohort study. Geriatric Orthopaedic Surgery and Rehabilitation. 2024;**15**:21514593241273124. DOI: 10.1177/21514593241273124

[17] Simunovic N, Devereaux PJ, Sprague S, Guyatt GH, Schemitsch E, DeBeer J, et al. Effect of early surgery after hip fracture on mortality and complications: Systematic review and meta-analysis. CMAJ Canadian Medical Association Journal. 2010;**182**:1609-1616. DOI: 10.1503/cmaj.092220

[18] Clegg A, Young J, Iliffe S, Rikkert MO, Rockwood K. Frailty in elderly people. The Lancet. 2013;**381**(9868):752-762. DOI: 10.1016/S0140-6736(12)62167-9

[19] Rockwood K, Mitnitski A. Frailty in relation to the accumulation of deficits. Journals of Gerontology - Series A Biological Sciences and Medical Sciences. 2007;**62**(7):722-727. DOI: 10.1093/gerona/62.7.722

[20] Liu W, Qin R, Qiu Y, Luan T, Qiu B, Yan K, et al. Multidimensional frailty as a predictor of mortality among older adults: A systematic review and meta-analysis. BMC Geriatrics. 2024;**24**:793

[21] Zanetti M, De Colle P, Niero M, Gortan Cappellari G, Barazzoni R, Ratti C, et al. Multidimensional prognostic index predicts short- and long-term mortality and rehospitalizations in older patients with hip fracture. Aging Clinical and Experimental Research. 2023;**35**(7):1487-1495. DOI: 10.1007/s40520-023-02433-8

[22] Hansen CM, Gadgaard NR, Vandenbroucke-Grauls C, Hailer NP, Pedersen AB. Interaction between multimorbidity and hip fracture surgery leads to excess risk of infection: A Danish registry-based cohort study of 92,599 patients with hip fracture. Clinical Epidemiology. 2025:167-176

[23] Veronese N, Ragusa FS, Hajek A, Stubbs B, Smith L, Barbagallo M, et al. Long-term impact of physical activity on mortality in adults with multimorbidity: A 12-year cohort longitudinal study from the survey on health, ageing and retirement in Europe. Journal of Cachexia, Sarcopenia and Muscle. 2025;**16**:e13695

[24] Ali A, Huszti E, Noordin S, Bogoch E, Yang A, Jain R, et al. The association between the number of chronic conditions and treatment of patients who are at high risk for future fracture in the Ontario fracture screening and prevention program (FSPP). Archives of Osteoporosis. 2025;**20**:28

[25] Switzer JA, O'connor MI. AAOS management of hip fractures in older adults evidence-based clinical practice guideline. JAAOS-Journal of the American Academy of Orthopaedic Surgeons. 2022;**30**:e1297-e1301

[26] Shen CY, Hsiao CH, Tsai W, Chang WH, Chen TH. Associations between hip fracture operation waiting time and complications in asian geriatric patients: A Taiwan medical center study. International Journal of Environmental Research and Public

Health. 2021;**18**(6):2848. DOI: 10.3390/ijerph18062848

[27] Lieten S, Herrtwich A, Bravenboer B, Scheerlinck T, Van Laere S, Vanlauwe J. Analysis of the effects of a delay of surgery in patients with hip fractures: Outcome and causes. Osteoporosis International. 2021;**32**(11):2235-2245. DOI: 10.1007/s00198-021-05990-8

[28] Bhatti UF, Shah AA, Williams AM, Biesterveld BE, Okafor C, Ilahi ON, et al. Delay in hip fracture repair in the elderly: A missed opportunity towards achieving better outcomes. Journal of Surgical Research. 2021;**266**:142-147. DOI: 10.1016/j.jss.2021.03.027

[29] Joseph EG, Serotte J, Haider MN, Pavlesen S, Anders M. Delay to surgical treatment in geriatric hip fracture patients. Geriatric Orthopaedic Surgery and Rehabilitation. 2023;**14**:1-8. DOI: 10.1177/21514593231204760

[30] Reider L, Furgiuele D, Wan P, Schaffler B, Konda S. Anesthetic methods for hip fracture. Current Osteoporosis Reports. 2024;**22**:96-104. DOI: 10.1007/s11914-023-00835-1

[31] Griffiths R, Babu S, Dixon P, Freeman N, Hurford D, Kelleher E, et al. Guideline by the association of anaesthetists: Guideline for the management of hip fractures 2020. Anaesthesia. 2021;**76**:225-237. DOI: 10.1111/anae.15291

[32] Konda SR, Solasz S, Ganta A, Egol KA. Monitored anesthesia care and soft tissue infiltration with local anesthesia: An anesthetic option for high-risk patients with hip fractures. Journal of Orthopaedic Trauma. 2023;**37**(8S):S3-S4. DOI: 10.1097/BOT.0000000000002635

[33] Yee DKH, Lau TW, Fang C, Ching K, Cheung J, Leung F. Orthogeriatric multidisciplinary co-management across acute and rehabilitation care improves length of stay, functional outcomes and complications in geriatric hip fracture patients. Geriatric Orthopaedic Surgery and Rehabilitation. 2022;**13**:1-15. DOI: 10.1177/21514593221085813

[34] De Vincentis A, Behr AU, Bellelli G, Bravi M, Castaldo A, Galluzzo L, et al. Orthogeriatric co-management for the care of older subjects with hip fracture: Recommendations from an Italian intersociety consensus. Aging Clinical and Experimental Research. 2021;**33**(9):2405-2443. DOI: 10.1007/s40520-021-01898-9

[35] Moppett IK, Parker M, Griffiths R, Bowers T, White SM, Moran CG. Nottingham hip fracture score: Longitudinal and multi-assessment. British Journal of Anaesthesia. 2012;**109**(4):546-550. DOI: 10.1093/bja/aes187

[36] Thorne G, Hodgson L. Performance of the Nottingham hip fracture score and clinical frailty scale as predictors of short and long-term outcomes: A dual-centre 3-year observational study of hip fracture patients. Journal of Bone and Mineral Metabolism. 2021;**39**(3):494-500. DOI: 10.1007/s00774-020-01187-x

[37] Wong RMY, Zu Y, Chau WW, Tso CY, Liu WH, Ng RWK, et al. High Charlson comorbidity index score is associated with early fracture-related complication for internal fixation of neck of femur fractures. Scientific Reports. 2022;**12**(1):4749. DOI: 10.1038/s41598-022-08855-0

[38] Nayak S, Singer A, Greenspan SL. Cost-effectiveness of secondary fracture prevention intervention for Medicare beneficiaries. Journal of the American

Geriatrics Society. 2021;**69**(12):3435-3444. DOI: 10.1111/jgs.17381

[39] Yu Y, Wang Y, Hou X, Tian F. Recent advances in the identification of related factors and preventive strategies of hip fracture. Frontiers in Public Health. 2023;**11**:1-15. DOI: 10.3389/fpubh.2023.1006527

[40] Min K, Beom J, Kim BR, Lee SY, Lee GJ, Lee JH, et al. Clinical practice guideline for postoperative rehabilitation in older patients with hip fractures. Annals of Rehabilitation Medicine. 2021;**45**(3):225-259. DOI: 10.5535/ARM.21110

[41] Handoll HHG, Cameron ID, Mak JCS, Panagoda CE, Finnegan TP. Multidisciplinary rehabilitation for older people with hip fractures. Cochrane Database of Systematic Reviews. 2021;**11**:CD007125, 1-193. DOI: 10.1002/14651858.CD007125.pub3

[42] Backman C, Harley A, Papp S, French-Merkley V, Beaulé PE, Poitras S, et al. Barriers and enablers to early identification, referral and access to geriatric rehabilitation post-hip fracture: A theory-based descriptive qualitative study. Geriatric Orthopaedic Surgery and Rehabilitation. 2022;**13**:1-22. DOI: 10.1177/21514593211047666

[43] Levy C, Ocampo-Chan S, Huestis L, Renzetti D. Early rehabilitation for patients with hip fractures: Spreading change across the system. Healthcare Quarterly. 2017;**20**(1):29-33. DOI: 10.12927/hcq.2017.25088

[44] Mattiazzo GF, Drewes YM, van Eijk M, Achterberg WP. Geriatric rehabilitation care after hip fracture. European Geriatric Medicine. 2023;**14**(2):295-305. DOI: 10.1007/s41999-023-00755-4

[45] Arkley J, Dixon J, Wilson F, Charlton K, Ollivere BJ, Eardley W. Assessment of nutrition and supplementation in patients with hip fractures. Geriatric Orthopaedic Surgery and Rehabilitation. 2019;**10**:1-7. DOI: 10.1177/2151459319879804

[46] Krakers SM, Woudsma S, van Dartel D, Vermeer M, Vollenbroek-Hutten MMR, Hegeman JH, et al. Rehabilitation of frail older adults after hip fracture surgery: Predictors for the length of geriatric rehabilitation stay at a skilled nursing home. Journal of Clinical Medicine. 2024;**13**:4547

Chapter 7

Making the Patient the Core of Nutritional Decision-Making (Oral Versus Tube Feeding): Surmounting Challenges amid Dysphagia and Life-Limiting Illness

Jennifer Hanners Gutierrez

Abstract

Overmedicalization of patients can occur in the context of critical or terminal illness. Tube feeding is a common recommendation for patients who desire nutrition and are diagnosed with dysphagia and life-limiting illness. Tube feeding has been found to cause harm in patients at the end of life without improving longevity. Oral feeding, such as careful hand feeding, has been found to better support psychosocial and physiological health. Past studies have reported lower incidence of pneumonia, depression, and mortality with oral feeding compared to tube feeding in persons with dysphagia and advanced dementia, stroke, or chronic obstructive pulmonary disease (COPD). Nutritional decision-making is an essential component of palliative care, and feeding routes must be weighed. Default use of tube feeding when a patient demonstrates difficulty swallowing is not supported by evidence. In addition, tube feeding should not be used to expedite treatment and transfer from a tertiary center to a facility that may potentially reap financial benefit from enteral versus oral nutrition. Research supports patient-centered care that focuses on shared decision-making, compassionate collaboration, skilled communication/documentation, and the upholding of a patient's right to choose a desired feeding route by informed autonomous consent.

Keywords: dysphagia, pneumonia, tube feeding, careful hand feeding, nutrition, oral versus tube feeding, palliative care, nutritional decision-making, end of life

1. Introduction

According to science, one's ability to eat and drink by mouth supports psychological [1] and physiological health. From the very beginning, infants bond with parents through nourishment and the associated intimacy/closeness that they experience during breast or bottle feeding. Throughout life and in elder-aged individuals, food is a connection to others and comfort [2]. Anatomical and muscular changes at the end

IntechOpen

of life combine with health care complications and often contribute to dysphagia (difficulty swallowing) [3]. Health care providers may react to dysphagia by withdrawing the option for oral nutrition due to feared consequences of tracheal and pulmonary aspiration (i.e., pathogens entering the airway by way of food or drink, increasing likelihood of a lung infection) [4]. It remains a widespread practice to replace oral nutrition with tube feeding with counsel that this type of feeding route is "safer." Past studies contradict this as related to dysphagia and terminal illness. In fact, recent research reports greater harm (pneumonia, depression, mortality) from use of tube feeding versus oral feeding when patients have dysphagia, desire nutrition, and are facing life-limiting illness [5, 6].

Moreover, theories have emerged from qualitative data that indicate the greater investment by health care providers, the greater chance for closure [7]. Yet, health care providers may make nutritional decisions based on their own biases, old research, or ease of discharge (e.g., place a tube and get the patient transferred out of the facility) [8]. Investment in biomedical ethics, shared decision-making [9], and patient-centered care needs further improvement so that patients may be offered well-grounded education and sound guidance when they want to eat by mouth with risk of aspiration.

As we move forward into an in-depth discussion regarding nutritional decision-making in the context of critical or life-limiting illness, consider two polar opposite case studies. The first patient had advanced-stage Parkinson's Disease. Due to this advanced progressive degenerative process, the patient was having trouble walking and intermittent coughing with oral feeding had begun. In addition, the patient began experiencing cardiac issues, and the surgeon decided to perform a complex heart surgery which resulted in a prolonged, worsened patient state. A speech-language pathologist was consulted to complete clinical and instrumental swallow examinations. Consistent aspiration was noted on a Modified Barium Swallow Study (videofluoroscopic swallow examination); therefore, the surgeon chose to schedule a percutaneous endoscopic gastrostomy (PEG) (i.e., placement of a stomach tube). The family communicated their disagreement with this procedure amid the patient's continued declining state. The physician team did not acknowledge the family's wishes, with nursing staff reporting that the primary physician "does not believe in palliative care or hospice." Ethical concerns arose and were addressed. The family acquiesced. The patient received a stomach tube. The patient did not wake up again for the remainder of his stay in the tertiary center, kept alive by chest tubes and supportive, high-volume oxygen and eventually transferred from the tertiary center prior to his passing.

In contrast, a patient was admitted to a tertiary center and diagnosed with an untreatable, progressive systemic (including throat) cancer with expected rapid decline and a terminal prognosis. The patient was unable to comfortably eat by mouth within a matter of days. The medical team consulted speech-language pathology to complete a clinical swallow examination. It was no longer comfortable for the patient to swallow. The patient became depressed and requested to "drink Coca-Cola™" while listening to George Strait. Oral swabs dipped in soda were offered to the patient to satisfy his craving while he listening to his favorite music artist. When a health care provider entered the room and asked what he was doing, he replied, "Drinking Coke and listening to George Strait." It is the first time in days he did not reply, "I'm dying," when asked how or what he was doing. No tube feeding was provided at his request. The patient was allowed to choose how he wanted to die.

These two case studies highlight the difference we can make as health care providers. We must weigh the feeding route and explore options that are evidenced-based and aligned with a patient's personal health care "story" and the patient's, or medical power of attorney's (MPOA's), wishes. It is the patient who governs care and, regardless of our years of medical training and good intentions, we are not able to make decisions independent of patient input. Patients, in many cases, may not want to sacrifice eating by mouth, citing food as: (a) dignity, (b) empowerment, (c) comfort, and (d) belonging [10].

2. Oral feeding versus tube feeding: An essential part of nutritional decision-making at the end of life

2.1 Why is food important?

Why is eating by mouth something that people/patients want to preserve? It is important, because food and drink are present at almost every momentous event in life—weddings, birthdays, celebrations, etc. When memories swell, they are almost never void of the laughter or tears that occurred while eating or drinking with loved ones. Past studies have revealed that when oral nutrition is withdrawn, psychosocial health suffers [1, 10]. Those who are no longer able to enjoy food or drink by mouth, but rather, are tube fed for nourishment experience social isolation and resulting depression.

Baumeister and Leary reported the innate human need to belong [11]. Our identity is a culmination of the groups to which we belong. For example, each of us may belong to several groups, such as groups related to church, sports, academia, work, family and more. When life events shift one's ability to stay connected to a group, one's identity may be disrupted. Mental health may suffer. The cessation of oral nutrition, replaced by tube feeding, changes the identity of a patient to one who can no longer socialize with family or friends through eating together. Friends may be lost, and family may no longer feel comfortable eating their food around a loved one who is unable to eat and drink by mouth. Meal times become quiet and depressing. Life changes.

Eating "normally" also provides a patient with greater dignity and, for as long as a patient can self-serve or eat with intermittent assistance (e.g., elbow support, hand-over-hand), a sense of empowerment remains. Careful hand oral feeding is an option when disease or injury progresses [12] and, although this requires the full assistance of the feeder, the meal can still be enjoyable as the feeder compassionately interacts with the patient, offering favorite flavors and foods.

Psychological health cannot be dismissed due to its impact on physiological health. When medical choices are made or unavoidable life circumstances occur that diminish psychosocial stability, physiological changes may result. A longitudinal study that compared psychological and physical health during pre-confinement and confinement during the Covid-19 pandemic found negative psychological *and* physical changes during the confinement period as compared to pre-pandemic states [13]. Lastly, Glannon [14] elucidated how stressful events can change physiology. Thus, changing someone's ability to eat by mouth, especially when a patient pleads for food and drink, may have consequences beyond sadness.

2.2 If tube feeding can cause problems, why is it used so often?

Dysphagia (difficulty swallowing) is a common reason that a health care provider may recommend that a patient receive nutrition via a tube versus by mouth. Problems with swallowing are the result of age combined with health care complications, such as stroke [15]. Dysphagia can also occur in younger patients as a result of disease or injury. Oropharyngeal dysphagia can be assessed clinically (e.g., at bedside) or instrumentally (e.g., fluoroscopically or endoscopically) and may include one or more of the following: (a) anterior loss of food or drink from the mouth (i.e., poor lip seal); (b) difficulty chewing; (c) prolonged anterior-to-posterior transport of food or drink; (d) oral residue or pocketing of food; (e) delayed pharyngeal engagement of swallow; (f) nasal regurgitation/poor velar movement, and (f) weak or deficient movement in swallowing musculature (e.g., laryngeal elevation, hyoid excursion, epiglottal inversion, pharyngeal and laryngeal constriction, pharyngeal stripping and clearance). Problems with swallowing can lead to entry of food or drink into the trachea (airway) and lungs. This can cause pneumonia which, in the context of life-limiting illness, can prompt patient decompensation due to acute respiratory compromise. Therefore, health care providers strive to avoid a climate that may contribute to aspiration pneumonia, often overmedicalizing through the use of tube feeding even when patients or MPOAs are willing to risk the consequences of eating and drinking by mouth amid dysphagia.

What kinds of health care complications worsen dysphagia? There are several life-limiting conditions that past studies have shown to be heavily associated with incidence of dysphagia. Dysphagia commonly occurs following traumatic brain injury (TBI), stroke, or progressive degenerative neural injury or disease process. Research has reported dysphagia to be present in over 70% of persons who have suffered a stroke, with 15% of patients with stroke and dysphagia having impressive problems after 6 months [16]. A separate study reported dysphagia present in 53% of patients admitted to a tertiary care center and post stroke [17]. Past studies have also shown the negative impact of a subdural hematoma (SDH) on swallowing with 13% of patients post SDH experiencing dysphagia [18]. Evidence reports SDH to account for over 50% of TBI. El Halabi et al. [19] reported dysphagia present in a vast array of neurogenic conditions including Myasthenia Gravis, Parkinson's Disease, and Amyotrophic Lateral Sclerosis (ALS).

Dysphagia is also frequently a complication of respiratory disease or instability. Li et al. [20] reported incidence of dysphagia in patients with Chronic Obstructive Pulmonary Disease (COPD) at 32.7%. Gastroesophageal Reflux Disease (GERD), dyspnea, and sputum bacteria were risk factors. Langmore et al. [21] reported dysphagia present in 33% of patients with acute respiratory failure and who required at least 48 hours of mechanical ventilation. Trauma also raises likelihood of dysphagia with research reporting dysphagia in 29% of patients following trauma, such as spinal cord injury (SCI) [22]. Mechanical ventilation increases the likelihood of complications related to trauma-related dysphagia.

Viral complications such as Human Immunodeficiency Virus (HIV) and Covid-19 are associated with dysphagia. Nustas et al. [23] reported dysphagia in 4.2% (8,699 of 206,332) of hospitalized persons diagnosed with HIV. Dysphagia increased length of hospital stay and rate of readmission within a 30-day period. Printza et al. [24] reported 63% of hospitalized patients admitted to an intensive care unit demonstrated dysphagia in association with Covid-19. Moreover, a 2023 retrospective analysis reported 55 out of 101 patients diagnosed with sepsis also experienced dysphagia [25].

Head and neck cancer has been reported to have a strong relationship to dysphagia. Kuhn et al. [26] constructed a consensus statement and reported dysphagia detected in 28% of new cancer presentations and in 75% of pharyngeal cancers.

Cristofaro et al. [27] reported weight loss and malnourishment as complications of patients with cancer and dysphagia, reporting 76% of the population with dysphagia presenting with severe malnutrition early in their course of care.

Lastly, kidney disease and liver disease have both been shown to have a relationship to dysphagia. Nativ-Zeltzer et al. [28] found kidney disease to be an independent risk factor for pneumonia in 698 patients diagnosed with dysphagia which was detected via instrumental testing. Chronic dysphagia (lasting more than 90 days) has also been found to be associated with advanced cirrhosis and endoscopic band ligation (EBL) [29].

Dysphagia, then, becomes a barrier to patients receiving food and drink due to health care providers recognizing the alignment of life-limiting diagnoses with swallowing problems and fearing patient harm from pulmonary aspiration. This presents significant challenges to health care providers who want to meet the psychological needs of patients while reducing suffering and preserving physiological health and comfort at the end of life. There are evidence-based ways to navigate dysphagia and feeding route when a patient desires nutrition (and pleads for oral nutrition) amid critical or terminal illness. First, let us ensure a full understanding of tube feeding (risks and benefits).

2.3 Tube feeding (risks and benefits)

Within the medical arena, there is a pervasive lack of knowledge about different enteral (tube) feeding options and why one option might be chosen over another. It is necessary to understand the differences between most commonly used enteral feeding methods if one is to be recommended [30]. It is also essential to understand that no method of tube feeding is risk free as related to tracheal and pulmonary aspiration.

When patients are diagnosed with dysphagia by the medical team based on clinical indicators of a swallowing problem or via analysis by a speech-language pathologist, a nasogastric (NG) tube may be recommended for nutrition. The nasogastric tube is radio-opaque and ranges from fine-bore (≤ 12 French) to wide-bore (>12 French). Larger bore sizes may be chosen for patients receiving medications that may clog smaller tubes. The NG tube is placed through the nose, down the esophagus, through the lower esophageal sphincter, and into the stomach. This method is often chosen when health care providers feel the swallowing problem may be short term. In a seminal, multicenter, randomized trial, researchers reported positive patient outcomes associated with early use of a NG following stroke [31]. There are challenges and risks, however. The NG is commonly placed in the patient's room. Although radio-opaque, nurses and health care providers are busy, and the NG is typically not placed using x-ray technology. This can result in misplacement (insertion into the lungs versus stomach) and can be life-threatening. There is also risk of perforation (e.g., esophageal perforation) in patients with fragile tissue and anatomical deviations [32]. Lastly, in patients with upper gastrointestinal abnormalities, there is likelihood of reflux and retrograde flow of liquid nutrition delivered by tube with increased risk of aspiration.

When medication administration via tube is not a concern and gastric decompression or drainage is not required, a Dobhoff tube may be an option. The Dobhoff tube is placed similar to the NG but is a smaller bore size. Due to the smaller French size, the Dobhoff tube may be more comfortable and less irritating to the esophagus. The Dobhoff tube may be placed into the stomach, and post-pyloric placement into the duodenum or jejunum is also possible which lessens risk of aspiration. Liu et al. [33]

conducted a meta-analysis, reviewing 41 studies conducted in 10 countries with over 3000 participants. It was discovered the post-pyloric enteral feeding lessened risk of pulmonary aspiration, gastric reflux, and pneumonia. One consideration with post-pyloric placement of a Dobhoff tube is nutrient absorption, as nutrients bypass the stomach's acidic environment and initial enzymatic activity, including limited gastric lipase for fat digestion and pepsin for protein breakdown. Although the majority of fat and protein digestion occurs in the small intestine, direct delivery to the jejunum may reduce exposure to bile and pancreatic enzymes when the tube is placed distal to the duodenum. Nonetheless, with strategic feeding protocols and improved enteral formulations, this has become less of a barrier to patient nourishment than it was historically.

Some patients are not expected to regain swallow functionality quickly or health care providers do not believe the patient can swallow "safe" enough to avoid long-term enteral feeding. Therefore, a gastrostomy tube (G-tube) is recommended. The stomach tube can be placed endoscopically (PEG), fluoroscopically, or surgically (open gastrostomy). As mentioned previously, a G-tube is typically viewed as a more permanent option; although, it can be removed if a patient's swallowing functionality improves. There is typically less likelihood of reflux with the G-tube, as it does not hold the lower esophageal sphincter open. However, reflux and aspiration of tube feeding can still occur in patients with GERD, gastroparesis, and alternative gastrointestinal abnormalities. Risk of infection, tube dislodgement, and abdominal discomfort have a stronger relationship to a G-tube than a NG tube or Dobhoff. Kohli et al. [34] used archival data analysis to determine comparative adverse event risk of each gastrostomy placement technique. Researchers discovered that there was significantly less risk of colon perforation, hemorrhage, or infection with PEG versus fluoroscopic or surgical placements.

Similar to a Dobhoff, a jejunostomy tube (J-tube) is an alternative option when long-term artificial nutrition and hydration (ANH) may be needed, and gastrointestinal concerns heighten risk of aspiration if enteral feeding is delivered to the stomach. The J-tube can be placed endoscopically, radiologically, or surgically. The J-tube is placed into the jejunum (i.e., the middle section of the small intestine). Risks include: (a) dislodgement, (b) infection, (c) bowel perforation, and (d) granulation tissue. These risks are similar to a G-tube; therefore, if a patient has increased odds of aspirating enteral feeding if delivered by G-tube, a J-tube lessens these odds and may be a reasonable choice. Conrad et al. [35] conducted a multi-institutional, retrospective study to determine patient outcomes as related to J-tube placement following diagnosis of esophageal cancer with esophagectomy. Patients who underwent J-tube placement had significantly improved nutritional outcomes and reduced 90-day mortality and recurrence rates.

Use of tube feeding has been found to improve patient outcomes in certain patient populations. Tube feeding may be beneficial in the context of oropharyngeal cancer. Anderson et al. [36] investigated tube feeding use and practices from 2015 to 2021 in a comprehensive cancer center. It was determined that 27% of patients diagnosed with oropharyngeal cancer received G-tubes. Li et al. [37] investigated feeding tube use in patients with esophageal cancer. Results revealed 38% (132/350) received a feeding tube and 50 out of the 132 had a reactive feeding tube placement due to severe dysphagia and a need for chemotherapy. There was greater incidence of complications in the group requiring reactive feeding tube placement, suggesting that earlier intervention as related to enteral feeding for patients with degraded swallow functionality and an aggressive treatment plan may be fruitful.

Tube feeding is used consistently to improve patient outcomes amid impressive wounds, such as burn injuries. In 2023, researchers reported enteral nutrition to be the preferred feeding route for patients following burn injury [38], citing a study by Mosier et al. [39] that reported fewer wound infections and shorter lengths of stay in the intensive care unit when early intervention with tube feeding was implemented. In addition, patients who receive tube feeding following TBI have good outcomes. Marshall et al. [40] reported benefits of early tube feeding (i.e., within 48 hours) and elucidated advantages, such as reduced inflammation, immunological response, and gastrointestinal health.

In contrast, tube feeding has been found to be associated with harm in persons with advanced-stage dementia, stroke, and COPD. Gillick [41] reported increased pneumonia and mortality in the context of advanced dementia and tube feeding in seminal research completed in 2000. Cintra et al. [6] conducted a prospective observational research study comparing patient outcomes as related to oral versus tube feeding in persons with dementia. Results revealed increased rates of aspiration pneumonia and mortality. Hanners Gutierrez et al. [5] completed an archival data analysis which analyzed patient outcomes based on feeding route (oral or tube) in patients diagnosed with dysphagia and end-stage stroke or end-stage COPD. Through propensity score analysis (i.e., in a matched dataset, randomized by algorithm), significant results were achieved. Researchers determined pneumonia to be 10.14 times more likely to occur amid tube feeding versus oral feeding. Depression was 2.79 times more likely to occur with tube feeding, and participants who were tube-fed versus oral-fed had 3.02 greater odds of mortality. A review by Elmahdi et al. in 2023 [42] listed dysphagia as a risk factor in patients who received tube feeding and suffered aspiration pneumonia and mortality. Associations of tube feeding to depression and infection in adult patients across diagnoses have been found in both restorative and palliative care climates.

3. Governors of nutritional decision-making: Ethical, legal, and clinical underpinnings

Many patients request to eat by mouth amid life-limiting illness. Evidence largely supports oral feeding with risk reduction strategies at the end of life versus enteral nutrition. What helps to govern our decisions as health care providers when encountering the challenge of managing nutrition at the end of life? Biomedical ethics, the World Health Organization's definition of palliative care, and the Patient Self Determination Act comprise the umbrella under which nutritional decision-making falls.

Biomedical ethical principles are as follows: (a) respect for patient autonomy, (b) beneficence, (c) non-maleficence, and (d) justice [43]. Having respect for patient autonomy means listening to your patient. However, it also means providing well-grounded evidence so that the patient or MPOA can make an informed choice. Health care providers must take care to provide information in a manner that excludes bias and offers current, sound, peer-reviewed/research-based guidance as to risks and benefits of a medical decision. Beneficence means "to do good." Health care providers likely have the best of intentions when recommending medical equipment or procedures; however, the long-term implications of a medical decision may not be considered when giving advice. For example, a wealth of literature has examined the impact of tube feeding amid advanced-stage dementia. At the end of life, patients with dementia may cease wanting food or drink. Family members often become distraught when this shift occurs, fearing painful starvation in their loved one. Physicians may be tempted to recommend a feeding tube to provide nourishment and calm the emotions of caregivers. Past evidence, however, reports greater harm from tube feeding in the context of end-stage dementia and no benefit to longevity [41].

Non-maleficence means "do no harm." Again, the long-term implications of a medical decision must be considered prior to implementing a significant change in medical equipment or to the plan of care. For example, without vetting social or family support, health care providers may recommend a G-tube for a patient with cognitive deficits and little assistance. Perhaps this feeding route could be beneficial if the climate in which it was recommended was one of ample support and care, including tube feeding administration and infection control. Without the patient's comprehensive understanding of feeding tube logistics and with no help, this type of patient may become a casualty of this decision through frequent hospital readmissions for infection or tube feeding aspiration. Finally, justice can be defined as fair and equitable treatment. Careful hand/assisted feeding must be offered to all those who need it, including patients with little-to-no family or caregiver support. In the current health care infrastructure, when staffing shortages plague facilities, problem-solving how to ensure patients who choose to eat orally with risk are provided equitable assistance to do so is essential.

Standing hand-in-hand with biomedical ethics is the World Health Organization's definition of palliative care which underscores reduction of suffering as the key component [44]. Ethical management of a patient's expressed desire to eat by mouth requires attempting to meet this need. When a patient begins to significantly decompensate and decline, meeting this need becomes even more challenging. Health care providers should strive to do "the most." Sometimes "the most" is a hamburger. Sometimes it is carefully hand fed pureed food and single sips of liquid. At the end of life, "the most" may be an oral swab laced with a favorite flavor (e.g., root beer) and dabbed on the tongue. Feeding strategies at the end of life may not offer ideal nutritional support; however, psychological support, such as the comfort of a favorite flavor, may be enough. Past research offers data that support voluntary fasting at the end of life as a comfortable, pleasant, and peaceful transition [45].

The Patient Self-Determination Act of 1991 gave patients the right to choose their medical care and to refuse medical equipment, interventions, or procedures with which they disagree. Physicians and alternative health care providers invest years into studying what may improve the medical states of their patients – how to heal, how to save, and how to positively impact patients' lives as related to their health. However, patients are not required to accept recommendations of health care providers. Patients may create an Advanced Directive, a legal document outlining a care plan amid critical or terminal illness. Even in the absence of an Advanced Directive, a patient has a voice and can dictate what happens to their body. There is no medical intervention that can be done without a patient's verbal or written consent. The problem is—most patients and many health care providers do not know this. This is why requiring a patient to change their code or care status (e.g., do not resuscitate [DNR], do not intubate [DNI], allow natural death [AND] and comfort care) to be able to have a sip of coffee amid dysphagia and risk of aspiration has not only ethical, but also legal, ramifications [46].

3.1 Navigating and surmounting barriers to oral feeding with risk at the end of life

One barrier to a patient being able to eat by mouth with risk is the fear of acute patient decline if the patient aspirates and requires cardiopulmonary resuscitation

(CPR). Physicians may want to support a patient's desire to eat and drink by mouth with risk, but they fear the outcome. This fear is understandable, and it elevates the importance of knowing evidence as related to aspiration risk with tube feeding (i.e., not risk free and can cause harm) and what strategies may be helpful as related to risk reduction if a patient chooses least risk oral feeding.

The rheology (property) of food can be modified. Different viscosities of food and drink pose varied degrees of aspiration risk. There may be benefits to changing a patient's diet in alignment with the International Dysphagia Diet Standardization Initiative (IDDSI): (a) liquid diet, (b) pureed, (c) minced and moist, (d) soft and bite sized, (e) easy-to-chew, and (f) regular. For example, softer, moldable viscosities are typically better tolerated by patients with oral motor weakness and an overall declining medical state that affects endurance and respiratory stability/support. Positioning is also a key component of eating with least risk. Patients diagnosed with dysphagia should eat and drink in an upright position, a side-lying position (to the stronger side if possible), or an inclined position/Reverse Trendelenburg as tolerated. There are times when a slightly reclined position may improve anterior-to-posterior bolus transport when patients with impressive lingual weakness struggle with this aspect of swallowing; the benefit of this position is best studied and practiced in the context of an instrumental swallow examination (e.g., modified barium swallow study [MBSS]).

Lastly oral care is one of best and underutilized techniques to inhibit pulmonary infection from aspiration [47]. Eliminating or reducing harmful bacteria in the mouth lessens the risk of pulmonary ingestion of oral pathogens (i.e., pathogens delivered to the lungs with food and drink that is aspirated). Patients with an elevated risk of aspiration should have routine oral care that may include tooth brushing (or denture cleaning) in the morning and at night and a gentle swab or swish with an evidenced-based solution after meals. Past research has reported diluted hydrogen peroxide [48] or chlorhexidine to be effective at reduction of harmful oral bacteria and ultimately protective of the lungs when pneumonia is a risk.

A second barrier to health care providers supporting least risk oral feeding is the fear of legal implications if a patient eats by mouth, aspirates, and experiences significant decline as a result. Some facilities require a patient or a MPOA to sign a waiver that acknowledges risk of aspiration if a patient chooses to eat by mouth. This waiver is used to "protect" the health care providers and the facility; however, there are problems with this [49]. A document such as this is only legally enforceable if both parties are on equal-ground. When a critically-ill patient is asked to sign a waiver by an authority figure, such as their primary physician, there is no equal ground so, by law, there is no legal protection offered by the waiver which is ultimately unenforceable in court. In addition, to my knowledge, there is no qualitative study that has reported a patient's desire to "choose death." A patient may choose reduction of suffering, perceived increased peace that may come amid the cessation of certain medical interventions, to go to Heaven or achieve spiritual closure, etc. Patients do not want to sign their name, however, officially stating that they are willing to die for food. There are evidence-based and effective strategies to use when discussing risks and benefits of medical decisions, such as feeding route. It is essential that health care providers do not bring shame to a patient who understands risks of a decision, expresses this understanding, but continues to plead for favorite foods. A waiver is understandable in theory but, by its very nature, can frighten or shame a patient into accepting an alternative feeding route that the patient has the right not to choose. How do health care providers surmount this barrier of fearing legal repercussions?

Communication and documentation is key to ensure that the patient or MPOA makes an informed autonomous choice and that shared decision-making is achieved.

3.2 Informed autonomous consent and the SPIKES protocol to ensure patient understanding of swallowing capability or lack thereof and to establish shared goals

A patient who wants to eat by mouth with risk of aspiration must choose this feeding route by informed autonomous consent [50]. This means that the patient (or MPOA) must wholly *understand* the implications of choosing this feeding route. The implications can be kindly discussed versus presenting risks void of compassion and understanding of what food means to a given patient. For example, a health care provider may say, "Mr. Jones, you have communicated that you are really missing your coffee. You and I have frequently discussed how sick you are, and I can see that you believe coffee may comfort you. Let's chat for a bit about what may happen if your coffee goes down the wrong way." Do not forget that beyond elucidating risks of oral feeding are the risks of tube feeding if a choice is offered to a patient or MPOA. Once sound evidence has been provided and risks and benefits disclosed, assessing the patient's understanding of this information is crucial. The patient or MPOA must *intend* to choose a particular feeding route. The health care provider must perceive clarity in whomever is making this choice; there can be no confusion. The patient or MPOA must *volunteer* the choice of feeding route. There can be no coercion. Research has shown that when a doctor or alternative health care provider enters the patient's room, that person is automatically seen as authoritative. Patients often do not believe they have a voice as related to their medical decisions; therefore, they tend to choose what the health care provider is perceived to want. This is why it is important to disconnect bias from informative discussions about feeding route. If the patient thinks YOU want it, they may choose it...even if it is not what is truly desired.

A physician or alternative health care provider who has fully disclosed what may happen as a result of a nutritional decision, confirmed patient or MPOA understanding [51], ensured the patient's intention to choose a particular feeding route, and prevented bias from influencing the patient's nutritional choice has met criteria for informed autonomous consent. The health care provider may document this consent as follows: "The patient wishes to eat by mouth with risk. Risks and benefits of alternative feeding routes were discussed at length, and the patient verbalized comprehensive understanding. The patient chooses least risk oral feeding by informed autonomous consent: (a) the patient intends to make this choice, (b) volunteers this choice, and (c) understands implications of this choice." Additional details of repeated discussion about feeding route(s) should also be included in chart notes/medical records.

The SPIKES Protocol began as a method of delivering bad news to oncology patients [52]. It is now being used throughout arenas of medicine as a template for hard conversations about health status and to guide both the health care provider and the patient in the context of a difficult decision. The first "S" stands for *Setting up* the interview. It is important to allow the patient to agree to a time to discuss a topic that may produce strong emotions, sadness, disappointment, etc. The health care provider should make a connection to the patient and strive to build rapport. Past evidence has reported the benefit of sitting down when holding a conversation with the patient [53]. When setting up the interview, strive to show compassion through soft skills (e.g., smiling, calm tone of voice) and find an item on which to sit. Make eye contact. Listen intently. The patient may agree to hold the conversation immediately, or the health care provider may be asked to return at a later time. The next step in the SPIKES Protocol is to assess the patient's *Perception*. It is essential that when discussing why a patient might choose a particular feeding route amid critical or terminal illness that the patient actually recognizes the gravity of their medical condition. A gentle approach works best. For example, "How do you feel about your current situation? Tell me your thoughts about how sick you have been recently?" If the oncology team has yet to educate the patient as related to the results of the biopsy, it may not be the time to directly state, "Your cancer is severe and will affect your ability to eat comfortably by mouth."

Once the patient's perception of their medical state is clear and accurate, it is appropriate to kindly request an *Invitation* to proceed with dispersion of *Knowledge* to help inform medical, nutrition decision-making. The health care provider should review swallow testing results and comprehensively cover risks and benefits of feeding route options. This is the stage of the SPIKES Protocol when information is outlined thoroughly to meet the criterion of patient understanding related to informed autonomous consent. The physician or alternative health care provider should show *Empathy* during the course of this informative conversation. Statements such as, "I understand," are typically not well received, as patients may wonder how a doctor can "understand" what it feels like to be dying. Instead, statements like, "I can see this is truly upsetting to you, and I am sorry," convey insight into the patient's current emotional state. Before the health care provider concludes a difficult conversation such as this, care should be taken to ensure a patient's full understanding of knowledge provided. An effective way to do this may be to simply ask, "Tell me your understanding of the things that you and I have discussed." The patient will likely have a surface understanding that the physician can improve through repetition of information or explaining details in a different manner.

Shared goals can be determined through a conversation led by the SPIKES blueprint. The health care provider should always know the goals of the patient. It does not make sense for the physician to potentially argue the risks of a hamburger when all the patient craves is a taste of Dr. Pepper. Once goals are established, the health care provider can explain how the plan of care is specifically designed to meet the expressed goals of the patient. Shared goals setting also presents an opportunity for the physician to express any misalignment between the plan of care and the patient's expressed goals. For example, the patient's goal may include complete resolution of pulmonary instability, but the patient chooses to eat orally with risk (when impressive aspiration has been detected on a swallowing examination). This presents a challenge. This challenge does not indicate that the patient must change the code status to be permitted oral nutrition. It also does not mean that the patient has no right to choose to eat by mouth with risk. It does mean, however, that the patient needs to understand the consequences of the choice. A situation like this challenges the physician to enact repeated, informative, compassionate conversations that encourage goal adjustment until a reasonable plan of care that meets the desires of the patient but supports physician intervention(s) or non-interventions is established.

4. Elevating "seeing" and investing in the patient

In considering palliative care patients' perspectives regarding plans of care as related to the best option for a feeding route (oral or tube), researchers have asked questions related to:

1. What is happening here?

2. What are the participants feeling?

3. What do the actions in this data show?

4. What is meaningful in this data?

5. What do they care about?

6. What explains the behaviors?

Investigations have revealed thematic behaviors patients use to prevent loss of control [54]. Resistance, anger, and protesting are common behaviors reported amid qualitative data analysis. These behaviors illustrate the painful experience of loss and represent *struggle for control*. Increased struggle for control appears to have a relationship to overall preparedness for patient death. When family members or loved ones are unprepared for patient death or unwilling to accept possibility of patient death, struggle ensues. Greater loss of control is perceived. Past research indicates that control, which may be partially defined as personal involvement in care and decision-making, is moderated by empowerment [55]. When a patient feels heard and decisions are made inclusively, there is a sense of control--even if all expressed desires are not met.

There are varying degrees of investment from medical providers. If investment moderates control, then medical providers must achieve a firm grasp of what investment looks like "in action." Past studies have found that *investment* includes advocacy, education, building relationships, spiritual support, and establishing a connection [56]. Effective investment includes application of knowledge and skill and "something beyond." What is "effective investment?" What is "beyond?" Effective investment may include: (a) believing in your patient, (b) showing interest, and (c) resisting barriers such as judgment or reacting negatively to patient resistance. A relationship must be built for a patient to trust provider inclusion in their most intimate life moments—dying is intimate. Therefore, it can be argued that entering a patient's room and "doing your job" is not enough. Simply asking about the patient's life can create trust needed to proceed with swallow analysis/nutritional decision-making, as can showing compassion for the patient's situation. In this sense, the medical provider becomes more than a provider, but rather, a coach and an advocate. Medical providers must be willing to speak up and be a "voice" for patients.

With critical illness, especially in Palliative Medicine, closure cannot mean "healed." *Closure* takes on a different meaning when discussing how a patient wants to live while severely-compromised and/or dying. It can be argued that greater clinical advocacy, education, relationship building, and investment lead to increased patient perception of control and closure evidenced by patient reports of peace and happiness. Field notes indicate several independent instances of a patient's "world having changed" following provision of oral nutrition at their request. Research has also revealed a relationship between closure and consensus on the nutritional decision amid medical providers, patients, and family members/caregivers. Does closure mean that oral nutrition is always the outcome? No, data do not support this; although, evidence points to many patients voicing a preference for oral alimentation [57]. Overall, successful closure occurs when the patient is able to contribute to or make an informed nutritional decision and is supported in doing so by health care providers who demonstrate excellent clinical skill, combined with clinical investment and patient empowerment. Consider a case study throughout which a patient indicated that he *was* ready to die. He just did not want to die being invisible—or without his coffee.

5. Conclusion

Nutritional decision-making is an essential and inevitable part of critical or terminal illness. Default use of tube feeding when patients have health care complications and dysphagia continues to be a common occurrence, even when patients request to eat and drink by mouth when dying. As health care providers, we have an obligation to use well-grounded evidence to weigh risks and benefits of feeding routes and to properly inform patients and caregivers. Health care providers are also obligated to listen to patients, to respond professionally and empathetically to their right to choose, and to meet criteria for informed autonomous choice of feeding route. Tube feeding should never be selected to expedite patient discharge, for perceived ease of medical interventions (e.g., bolus tube versus careful hand oral feeding), or for profit (e.g., research has reported fiscal incentives for nursing homes if residents are tube-fed) [58].

Tube feeding has been reported to cause harm to patients at the end of life versus providing a safer alternative for nutritional support, the driving force behind its frequent historic use and advocacy. In many cases, the harm is accompanied by no increase in or benefit to longevity. Therefore, rejecting a palliative care patient's pleas to eat and drink by mouth in the name of "safety" is not supported by evidence. While tube feeding has its place and can benefit patients, especially in the context of restorative care, its overuse needs to be curbed and the narrative surrounding its elimination of aspiration risk needs to stop. Proven methods of communicating risks and benefits as related to feeding route should be used and documentation should include description of efforts to fully disclose risks and benefits while ensuring the patient's or MPOA's comprehensive understanding of this information. Physician and health care provider alignment related to nutritional decision-making and collective investment in this aspect of comfort at the end of life is crucial to patients' psychological and physiological care.

Acknowledgements

The author would like to acknowledge the support of her work by Texas Tech University Health Sciences Center (TTUHSC) and UMC Health System in Lubbock, Texas, USA. In addition, the support of her Department Chair (Department of Otolaryngology in the TTUHSC School of Medicine), Dr. Joehassin Cordero, has been invaluable to the author's success. Lastly, the author would like to thank the TTUHSC Institutional Review Board and the Clinical Research Institute for their steadfast collaboration and assistance.

Author details

Jennifer Hanners Gutierrez
Texas Tech University Health Sciences Center and UMC Health System, Lubbock, Texas, USA

*Address all correspondence to: jennifer.hanners-gutierrez@ttuhsc.edu; gutierrez.speechpathology@outlook.com

References

[1] Hepper EC, Wilson J, Drinnan M, Patterson JM. Psychosocial impacts of being nil-by-mouth as an adult: A scoping review. Journal of Advanced Nursing. 2024;**80**(9):3499-3515

[2] Morley C. No Love Like It: Feeding Someone Who Is Sick. Altona, Canada: Friesen Press; 2025

[3] Thiyagalingam S, Kulinski AE, Thorsteinsdottir B, Shindelar KL, Takahashi PY. Dysphagia in older adults. In: Mayo Clinic Proceedings. Vol. 96. Elsevier; 2021. pp. 488-497

[4] Wilkinson JM, Codipilly DC, Wilfahrt RP. Dysphagia: Evaluation and collaborative management. American Family Physician. 2021;**103**(2):97-106

[5] Hanners Gutierrez J, Lazarus C, Corwin M, Leslie P. Pneumonia, depression, and mortality are impacted by feeding route in patients with dysphagia. Gerontology and Geriatric Medicine. 2024;**10**:1-8

[6] Cintra MT, de Rezende NA, de Moraes EN, Cunha LC, da Gama Torres HO. A comparison of survival, pneumonia, and hospitalization in patients with advanced dementia and dysphagia receiving either oral or enteral nutrition. The Journal of Nutrition, Health, and Aging. 2014;**18**(10):894-899

[7] Kuipers SJ, Nieboer AP, Cramm JM. Making care more patient centered; experiences of healthcare professionals and patients with multimorbidity in the primary care setting. BMC Family Practice. 2021;**22**:1-5

[8] Gumaste VV, Bhamidimarri KR, Bansal R, Sidhu L, Baum J, Walfish A. Factors predicting early discharge and mortality in post-percutaneous endoscopic gastrostomy patients. Annals of Gastroenterology. 2014;**27**(1):42-47

[9] O'Keeffe ST, Leslie P, Lazenby-Paterson T, McCurtin A, Collins L, Murray A, et al. Informed or misinformed consent and use of modified texture diets in dysphagia. BMC Medical Ethics. 2023;**24**(1):1-12

[10] Pizzorni N. Social and psychologic impact of dysphagia. In: Dysphagia: Diagnosis and Treatment. Cham: Springer International Publishing; 2017. pp. 873-886

[11] Baumeister RF, Leary MR. The need to belong: Desire for interpersonal attachments as a fundamental human motivation. Interpersonal Development. 2017;**30**:57-89

[12] Yuen JK, Chan FH, Chan TC, Chow DT, Chu SW, Shea YF, et al. Hospital careful hand feeding program reduced feeding tube use in patients with advanced dementia. The Journal of Nutrition, Health & Aging. 2023;**27**(6):432-437

[13] Fernández-Abascal EG, Martín-Díaz MD. Longitudinal study on affect, psychological well-being, depression, mental and physical health, prior to and during the COVID-19 pandemic in Spain. Personality and Individual Differences. 2021;**172**:1-10

[14] Glannon W. The psychology and physiology of depression. Philosophy, Psychiatry, & Psychology. 2002;**9**(3):265-269

[15] Labeit B, Michou E, Hamdy S, Trapl-Grundschober M, Suntrup-Krueger S, Muhle P, et al. The assessment

of dysphagia after stroke: State of the art and future directions. The Lancet Neurology. 2023;**22**(9):858-870

[16] Qin Y, Tang Y, Liu X, Qiu S. Neural basis of dysphagia in stroke: A systematic review and meta-analysis. Frontiers in Human Neuroscience. 2023;**17**:1-13

[17] Chacko SP, Joshi AA, Sangle VR, Arora DS, Dubey RA. Incidence of dysphagia in acute stroke patients: An early screening and management. Management. 2021;**11**(2):50-53

[18] Won SY, Krieger S, Dubinski D, Gessler F, Behmanesh B, Freiman TM, et al. Neurogenic dysphagia in subdural hematoma. Frontiers in Neurology. 2022;**12**:1-7

[19] El Halabi M, Arwani R, Parkman HP. Dysphagia in neurological disorders. In: Seminars in Neurology. Thieme Medical Publishers, Inc.; 2023. pp. 530-539

[20] Li W, Gao M, Liu J, Zhang F, Yuan R, Su Q, et al. The prevalence of oropharyngeal dysphagia in patients with chronic obstructive pulmonary disease: A systematic review and meta-analysis. Expert Review of Respiratory Medicine. 2022;**16**(5):567-574

[21] Langmore SE, Krisciunas GP, Warner H, White SD, Dvorkin D, Fink D, et al. Abnormalities of aspiration and swallowing function in survivors of acute respiratory failure. Dysphagia. 2021;**36**:831-841

[22] Freeman-Sanderson A, Crisp J, Hodgson CL, Holland AE, Harrold M, Chan T, et al. Prevalence, recovery, and factors associated with dysphagia in an older critically ill trauma cohort: A cross-sectional study. Australian Critical Care. 2024;**37**(6):957-963

[23] Nustas R, Dalsania R, Brown J, Patnana SV, Qayed E. Effect of dysphagia on hospital outcomes and readmissions in patients with human immunodeficiency virus. Southern Medical Journal. 2021;**114**(11):692-696

[24] Printza A, Tedla M, Frajkova Z, Sapalidis K, Triaridis S. Dysphagia severity and management in patients with COVID-19. Current Health Sciences Journal. 2021;**47**(2):147-156

[25] Hongo T, Yumoto T, Naito H, Fujiwara T, Kondo J, Nozaki S, et al. Frequency, associated factors, and associated outcomes of dysphagia following sepsis. Australian Critical Care. 2023;**36**(4):521-527

[26] Kuhn MA, Gillespie MB, Ishman SL, Ishii LE, Brody R, Cohen E, et al. Expert consensus statement: Management of dysphagia in head and neck cancer patients. Otolaryngology–Head and Neck Surgery. 2023;**168**(4):571-592

[27] Cristofaro MG, Barca I, Ferragina F, Novembre D, Ferro Y, Pujia R, et al. The health risks of dysphagia for patients with head and neck cancer: A multicentre prospective observational study. Journal of Translational Medicine. 2021;**19**:1-8

[28] Nativ-Zeltzer N, Nachalon Y, Kaufman MW, Seeni IC, Bastea S, Aulakh SS, et al. Predictors of aspiration pneumonia and mortality in patients with dysphagia. The Laryngoscope. 2022;**132**(6):1172-1176

[29] Idalsoaga F, Díaz LA, Ayares G, Cabrera D, Chahuan J, Monrroy H, et al. Oesophageal disorders in chronic liver disease. Alimentary Pharmacology & Therapeutics. 2024;**60**(6):715-726

[30] Reddick CA, Greaves JR, Flaherty JE, Callihan LE, Larimer CH, Allen SA.

Choosing wisely: Enteral feeding tube selection, placement, and considerations before and beyond the procedure room. Nutrition in Clinical Practice. 2023;**38**(2):216-239

[31] FOOD Trial Collaboration. Effect of timing and method of enteral tube feeding for dysphagic stroke patients (FOOD): A multicentre randomised controlled trial. The Lancet. 2005;**365**(9461):764-772

[32] Motta AP, Rigobello MC, Silveira RC, Gimenes FR. Nasogastric/nasoenteric tube-related adverse events: An integrative review. Revista Latino-Americana de Enfermagem. 2021;**29**:1-23

[33] Liu Y, Wang Y, Zhang B, Wang J, Sun L, Xiao Q. Gastric-tube versus post-pyloric feeding in critical patients: A systematic review and meta-analysis of pulmonary aspiration-and nutrition-related outcomes. European Journal of Clinical Nutrition. 2021;**75**(9):1337-1348

[34] Kohli DR, Kennedy KF, Desai M, Sharma P. Safety of endoscopic gastrostomy tube placement compared with radiologic or surgical gastrostomy: Nationwide inpatient assessment. Gastrointestinal Endoscopy. 2021;**93**(5):1077-1085

[35] Conrad H, Elkamel A, Maltagliati A, Wang K, Hsu CH, Linville W, et al. Outcomes of Jejunostomy tube placement in surgical patients with esophageal cancer. JTCVS Open. 2025;**24**:496-509

[36] Anderson BJ, Moreno AC, Qing Y, Lee JJ, Johnson FM, Lango MN, et al. Revisiting feeding tube utilization in oropharynx cancer: 6-year prospective registry analysis. Otolaryngology–Head and Neck Surgery. 2024;**170**(5):1319-1330

[37] Li Y, Pond G, Van Osch A, Reed R, Ung Y, Cheng S, et al. Enhancing nutrition support for esophageal cancer patients: Understanding factors influencing feeding tube utilization. Nutrition and Cancer. 2024;**76**(3):271-278

[38] Shields BA, Nakakura AM. Nutrition considerations for burn patients: Optimizing recovery and healing. European Burn Journal. 2023;**4**(4):537-547

[39] Mosier MJ, Pham TN, Klein MB, Gibran NS, Arnoldo BD, Gamelli RL, et al. Early enteral nutrition in burns: Compliance with guidelines and associated outcomes in a multicenter study. Journal of Burn Care & Research. 2011;**32**(1):104-109

[40] Marshall WA, Adams LM, Weaver JL. The brain–gut Axis in traumatic brain injury: Implications for nutrition support. Current Surgery Reports. 2022;**10**(10):172-179

[41] Gillick MR. Rethinking the role of tube feeding in patients with advanced dementia. New England Journal of Medicine. 2000;**342**(3):206-210

[42] Elmahdi A, Eisa M, Omer E. Aspiration pneumonia in enteral feeding: A review on risks and prevention. Nutrition in Clinical Practice. 2023;**38**(6):1247-1252

[43] Varkey B. Principles of clinical ethics and their application to practice. Medical Principles and Practice. 2021;**30**(1):17-28

[44] World Health Organization. Definition of palliative care. 2022. Available from: http://www.who.int/cancer/palliative/definition/en/

[45] Winter SM. Terminal nutrition: Framing the debate for the withdrawal of nutritional support in terminally

ill patients. The American Journal of Medicine. 2000;**109**(9):723-726

[46] Weaver MS, Geppert CM. Sometimes a difficult decision to swallow: Ethical dilemmas when patients with dysphagia who lack capacity want to eat. Journal of Pain and Symptom Management. 2023;**65**(1):97-102

[47] Scannapieco FA. Poor oral health in the etiology and prevention of aspiration pneumonia. Clinics in Geriatric Medicine. 2023;**39**(2):257-271

[48] Nobahar M, Razavi MR, Malek F, Ghorbani R. Effects of hydrogen peroxide mouthwash on preventing ventilator-associated pneumonia in patients admitted to the intensive care unit. Brazilian Journal of Infectious Diseases. 2016;**20**:444-450

[49] Horner J, Modayil M, Chapman LR, Dinh A. Consent, refusal, and waivers in patient-centered dysphagia care: Using law, ethics, and evidence to guide clinical practice. American Journal of Speech-Language Pathology. 2016;**25**(4):453-469

[50] Leslie P, Casper M. Ethical challenges: Less about moral wrongdoing and more about communication breakdown. Perspectives on Gerontology. 2015;**20**(3):72-84

[51] Millum J, Bromwich D. Informed consent: What must be disclosed and what must be understood? The American Journal of Bioethics. 2021;**21**(5):46-58

[52] Baile WF, Buckman R, Lenzi R, Glober G, Beale EA, Kudelka AP. SPIKES—A six-step protocol for delivering bad news: Application to the patient with cancer. The Oncologist. 2000;**5**(4):302-311

[53] Watts E, Patel H, Kostov A, Kim J, Elkbuli A. The role of compassionate care in medicine: Toward improving patients' quality of care and satisfaction. Journal of Surgical Research. 2023;**289**:1-7

[54] Black A, McGlinchey T, Gambles M, Ellershaw J, Mayland CR. The 'lived experience' of palliative care patients in one acute hospital setting–a qualitative study. BMC Palliative Care. 2018;**17**:1-10

[55] Wang R, Zhou C, Wu Y, Sun M, Yang L, Ye X, et al. Patient empowerment and self-management behaviour of chronic disease patients: A moderated mediation model of self-efficacy and health locus of control. Journal of Advanced Nursing. 2022;**78**(4):1055-1065

[56] McCaffrey N, Bradley S, Ratcliffe J, Currow DC. What aspects of quality of life are important from palliative care patients' perspectives? A systematic review of qualitative research. Journal of Pain and Symptom Management. 2016;**52**(2):318-328

[57] Santos CG, Mendes EC, Schramm FR, Costa MF. Oral feeding in oncologic palliative care. Revista Brasileira de Cancerologia. 2025;**70**:1-9

[58] Schneider PL, Fruchtman C, Indenbaum J, Neuman E, Wilson C, Keville T. Ethical considerations concerning use of percutaneous endoscopic gastrostomy feeding tubes in patients with advanced dementia. The Permanente Journal. 2021;**25**:1-5

Chapter 8

Intermittent Fasting in Geriatric Nutrition

Hilal Demirci

Abstract

The importance of nutrition for a healthy and long life is indisputable. People's nutritional routines are as important as their nutritional content. Instead of eating at fixed and unstable hours, eating routines limited to certain hours are a way of eating that suits metabolism and the circadian rhythm. Intermittent fasting, whose many benefits have been proven by studies, triggers autophagy, which detoxifies damaged organelles in cells. It reduces insulin resistance and metabolic syndrome by increasing insulin sensitivity. It has a positive effect on the lipid profile by increasing fatty acid oxidation. It reduces inflammation and has a neuroprotective effect that lowers the risk of neurodegenerative diseases. Intermittent fasting creates routines that restrict eating to varying intervals, such as 12 hours of fasting and 12 hours of eating, or 14–10, 16–8 hours, depending on the person and their health condition. Cellular detoxification becomes even more important with intermittent feeding due to the significant decrease in cellular production and repair in adults and geriatric individuals. Aging is inevitable; however, this process can be slowed down by the biochemical and visible effects of intermittent fasting on the body. It helps cells stay biologically young by providing them with the opportunity to renew themselves regularly. In this chapter, the effects of intermittent fasting, which begins in young and adult ages and continues into the geriatric period, on body metabolism will be examined.

Keywords: geriatric nutrition, metabolism, intermittent fasting, autophagy, cell regeneration

1. Introduction

The desire for longevity, which has developed around the myth of immortality throughout known history, has led to efforts in modern medicine to unravel the biology of aging and the mechanism of longevity. The desire for long life, which has developed around the myth of immortality throughout known history, has given way to efforts to unravel the mechanism of aging biology and longevity in today's modern medicine. The fact that the level of healthy aging has not increased at the same rate while life expectancy has been extended has become one of the greatest paradoxes of the world of medical science. This process is a complex biological phenomenon proven by medical indicators, in which metabolic, environmental, genetic and epigenetic factors play a role. This phenomenon has been tried to be elucidated by scientists through many scientific studies. In this study, the pathophysiological mechanisms underlying aging, which is not only a chronological event but also the sustainable lifestyle patterns that can be modified throughout the aging process, especially the time-restricted intermittent fasting (IF) model, which is a nutritional model, will be discussed. The IF nutritional model, whose potential benefits in geriatric nutrition are also being understood by gerontologists and can lead to a sustainable lifestyle, will be examined in the light of scientific clinical studies regarding its effects on many physiological mechanisms, especially autophagy, and its place in the geriatric population.

2. Physiology and theories of aging

Aging results from structural and functional changes that accumulate cumulatively throughout an organism's life at the cellular, tissue and organ levels. It is a natural process that cannot be avoided and is characterized by a decrease in the organism's capacity to maintain homeostasis, a decrease in resistance to diseases and an increase in the risk of death. Aging is characterized at the cellular level by DNA damage, telomere shortening, slowing cell division and mitochondrial dysfunction. Along with these, DNA mutations, free radical damage, lipid and protein oxidation occur in the organism. Due to the systemic changes that develop as a result of these, consequences such as susceptibility to chronic diseases, cognitive decline and decreased physical capacity occur. These systemic changes include impaired hormonal homeostasis, weakened immunity and decreased muscle and bone mass. And with these physiological steps, the organism enters the aging process, which is an inevitable end [1, 2].

In recent years, the elderly population around the world has increased significantly, and this increase is expected to accelerate in the coming decades. Between 2015 and 2030, the number of individuals aged 60 and over is projected to increase by 58%, from 910 million to 1.5 billion. By 2050, the global elderly population is expected to more than double, reaching almost 2.2 billion [3].

With the rapid increase in the world population and the significant increase in the number of individuals in the geriatric age group, an increase in the average life expectancy of people is also observed. The aging process of the world's population is progressing in the same and irreversible way at every point. This condition has profound medical and non-medical implications. The proportion of elderly individuals has reached its highest level in history and continues to increase worldwide. Since it is predicted that this situation will not change in the future, its important effects on health need to be addressed in detail [4].

In line with this prediction, health scientists have tried to solve the physiology of aging for many years in the light of developing science, and have tried to prevent cellular, metabolic and systemic aging and developed different hypotheses for humanity, which expects a long and healthy life.

One of the most notable among these is the free radical hypothesis. According to this hypothesis, free radicals, such as reactive oxygen species, formed during metabolic activities cause oxidative damage to macromolecules such as proteins, DNA and lipids and the cumulative accumulation of this damage over the years accelerates the aging process and leads to the death of the organism [5]. However, studies in recent years have suggested alternative approaches to explain the complex biological processes underlying aging.

DOI: http://dx.doi.org/10.5772/intechopen.1010918

This theory, called hormesis, is particularly used to explain the longevity effects caused by some nutraceutical compounds. Hormesis describes the activation of protective defense mechanisms at the cellular level as a result of organisms being exposed to low-level environmental stressors. These adaptive responses may provide a variety of biological benefits, such as modification of gene expression, regulation of metabolic processes and strengthening of antioxidant systems, thus ensuring both long and healthy life [5]. Thus, studies carried out to ensure healthy and long aging are developing nutrition-based interventions that can regulate metabolic homeostasis and stress levels [6].

3. Metabolic diseases and nutritional patterns in the aging process

Studies emphasizing nutritional interventions show that healthy aging is not a process limited to genetic inheritance but is directly related to the individual's lifestyle and nutritional habits. The three main factors contributing to healthy aging can be summarized as follows: (1) genetics and family history, (2) lifestyle and physical activity level and (3) diet and nutrition. Although genetics and family history cannot be changed, health status can be improved by optimizing lifestyle and nutritional habits with individual effort [7].

When we look at the diseases and deaths that develop under the influence of these basic factors that are essential for a healthy life, it is estimated that approximately 50 million people lose their lives each year in the world. The leading causes of global mortality are ischemic heart diseases (6.3 million deaths), cerebrovascular diseases (4.5 million deaths), lower respiratory tract infections (4.3 million deaths) and perinatal deaths (2.4 million deaths). In addition, COPD (2.2 million deaths), TB (2.0 million deaths), childhood rash diseases (1.2 million) and pulmonary CA (1 million deaths) are also among the leading causes of death [8]. The incidence and ease of these diseases are much higher in the geriatric period.

In addition to these diseases, the impact of nutrition-related diseases on global mortality rates in developed and developing countries is remarkable. In this context, the main diseases and disorders in which nutrition and lifestyle can play a protective role are hypertension and stroke, dyslipidemia and cardiovascular diseases, cancers, type 2 diabetes, sedentary life and obesity, musculoskeletal system diseases, osteoporosis, alzheimer's and other neuronal diseases. Preventive and therapeutic nutritional approaches, especially in elderly individuals, are of critical importance for public health [8].

It has been proven by many studies that healthy eating habits, which should be continued in adolescence and adulthood and into the geriatric period, can provide protection against diseases. In this context, many healthy eating patterns and diet recommendations covering all age groups have been developed. When geriatric age groups are examined; in addition to the requirements for macro and micro nutrients, the frequency and timing of meals have a direct effect on blood glycemic control, cardiovascular stability, gastrointestinal system functions and neurocognitive processes. Particularly in terms of comorbidities frequently seen in the geriatric age group, the creation of an individual-specific medical nutrition regimen plays a critical role in slowing down the progression of diseases and preventing complications. For this reason, nutrition in geriatric individuals should be evaluated not only in terms of calories and nutritional value, but also in terms of temporal organization and rhythmic structure.

When the relationship between healthy living and nutrition is examined in detail in the studies conducted, it is noteworthy that the rates of improvement in various metabolic diseases are significant. These disorders, grouped under the name of metabolic syndrome, are a clinical condition characterized by the coexistence of metabolic risk factors, according to the definition of the International Diabetes Federation, the American Heart Association and the National Heart, Lung and Blood Institute. And it is defined by the presence of at least three of the components. These are: central obesity, dyslipidemia, high blood pressure, impaired glucose metabolism and low level of high-density lipoprotein cholesterol (HDL). Metabolic syndrome has reached epidemic proportions, with an incidence of up to 25% in the adult population in developed countries [9–11]. Metabolic syndrome causes a 2-fold increase in the onset of type 2 diabetes and a 5-fold increase in the risk of major cardiovascular events, while provoking the development of diseases such as neurodegenerative diseases, circulatory disorders and cancer. This is the main problem of the adult population and poses a high threat to the health of the geriatric population [11].

The medical world has developed different nutrition and diet models by focusing on lifestyle and eating habits that have been proven to be effective in treating metabolic diseases, as they are both the main cause of mortality and morbidity and a major economic burden on the health system [9–11]. The main nutritional models whose effects and benefits on metabolism have been proven by scientific studies can be listed as follows.

Mediterranean diet (MedDiet): A nutritional model consisting mainly of plants, using cold-pressed extra virgin olive oil as a source of energy and fat, containing mostly vegetables, especially green leafy plants, legumes, fruits, whole grains and nuts. In traditional formulations of the diet, sauces called "sofrito" prepared with ingredients such as garlic, onion, olive oil and tomatoes have an important place. Such components are rich in biologically active phenolic compounds and carotenoids such as hydroxytyrosol, lycopene, naringenin and β-carotene, which contribute to the anti-inflammatory, antioxidant and cardioprotective effects of the diet [12].

Beyond the metabolic benefits provided by unsaturated fatty acids, high consumption of fruits and vegetables, which is one of the basic elements of the Mediterranean diet, supports the intake of bioactive components including antioxidant vitamins (e.g., vitamin C, vitamin E and β-carotene), phytochemical compounds such as polyphenols, folates and various elements. These components may have protective effects on various pathophysiological mechanisms such as reducing oxidative stress, modulating inflammation and supporting repair processes at the cellular level [13, 14].

In adults and geriatric individuals with high levels of compliance with the Mediterranean diet, a reduced prevalence and mortality of various chronic diseases, including cardiovascular diseases, malignant neoplasms and neurodegenerative diseases, has been observed [15, 16]. Numerous prospective cohort studies and randomized controlled trials have demonstrated that the MedDiet application provides clinically significant risk-reducing effects, particularly on the incidence of cerebrovascular events and cardiovascular events [17]. Mediterranean diet significantly reduced the severity of disease and complications in individuals diagnosed with metabolic diseases [13, 15].

Dietary approaches to stop hypertension (DASH) Diet: This nutritional model is designed specifically for blood pressure control in hypertensive individuals. It encourages consumption of mostly vegetables, fruits, whole grains, low-fat and nonfat dairy products, legumes and nuts, while limiting consumption of red and processed meat products and sugary drinks. The DASH diet has a low-fat content, providing approximately 25% of total energy intake from fat and the proportion of energy coming from saturated fat is around 6–7%. Dietary cholesterol is limited to 150 mg per day. Additionally, while sodium content is kept in the range of 1500–2250 mg/day, it is notable for its higher dietary fiber (>30–35 g/day), potassium, magnesium and calcium content compared to other dietary models [18, 19].

A meta-analysis of 31 randomized controlled trials evaluating the effectiveness of the DASH diet in the management of hypertension found that the use of this dietary pattern in combination with lifestyle changes resulted in significant reductions in systolic and diastolic blood pressure levels compared to individuals in the control group. In addition, it has been observed that as individual compliance with the DASH diet increases, the risk of developing metabolic syndrome decreases by approximately 50% due to decreases in body mass index (BMI), blood glucose levels and central obesity [20].

Low-carbohydrate diet: Low-carbohydrate diets are defined as diet models in which less than 50% of daily energy intake is provided by carbohydrates. These diets include limiting the consumption of processed foods, foods with added sugars, refined grains and starch sources, which are often bulky [21].

It is suggested that very low-carbohydrate ketogenic diets, which are generally less than 10% of total daily energy intake provided by carbohydrates (35–45 grams/day), may have the potential to improve the management of various chronic diseases such as overweight, obesity, cardiovascular diseases (CVD) and metabolic syndrome [22]. In this diet model, while the carbohydrate ratio is significantly reduced, fat consumption is significantly increased (fat/carbohydrate and protein ratio 3:1–4:1) [23]. Such restrictive dietary protocols have been associated with a decrease in body weight and an improvement in lipid profile, thus suggesting that they may have protective effects against obesity and CVD [22, 24]. However, it should be taken into consideration that the ketogenic diet may be insufficient for the balanced nutrients targeted in geriatric nutrition. In addition to the challenges encountered on a ketogenic diet, the potential negative effects of limited consumption of foods containing macro and micronutrients, such as fruits, vegetables and whole grain products, should be considered.

Among the nutritional models that can contribute to a long and healthy life, there are models that have not been studied sufficiently or that have not been proven to have a significant potential to improve metabolic disorders in the geriatric population, and whose continued safe use in the geriatric population is debatable. These dietary models are based on significant restriction of basic energy sources, especially those independent of macro and micronutrient distribution. These are; some plant-based diets, low-fat diets, high-protein diets, Nordic diet, etc. Most scientific evidence shows that in the management of metabolic diseases, it is the quality of macro and micronutrients consumed and the continuity of compliance with the diet rather than the quantity of nutrients in the diet that is important [25].

For many years, the importance of eating periods and patterns, as well as nutritional content, has been emphasized in the diet. In recent years, alternative nutrition models have come to the fore to slow down the aging process, support healthy aging and prevent chronic diseases. Among these models, calorie-restricted nutrition (CR) and intermittent fasting (IF) are particularly noteworthy. These approaches are widely included in studies due to their metabolic benefits, such as not only weight management but also delaying cellular aging, increasing insulin sensitivity and reducing inflammation. The evaluation of these nutritional models in terms of their applicability and effects on geriatric individuals is currently being researched by gerontologists and many scientists. Informing older people about individualized nutritional approaches not only provides a practical and economical solution, but also contributes to increasing holistic well-being by supporting physical, cognitive health and quality of life [26].

CR: Among the limited number of nonpharmacological therapeutic interventions investigated to improve age-related metabolic functions, Calorie restriction (CR) has been shown to reduce caloric intake without causing malnutrition, slowing the aging process and improving metabolic health. One of the CR studies conducted on humans, the Long-Term Effects of Reduced Caloric Intake Evaluation (CALERI-E) study, showed that there was limited weight loss, decreased daily energy expenditure and decreased levels of inflammation markers (Tumor Necrosis Factor) TNF-α and C-reactive protein (CRP) [27]. Many clinical studies have proven the benefits of CR on human health over the years and have shown weight loss and metabolic improvement after short- and long-term CR diet [28]. However, given the challenges of implementing and maintaining this dietary pattern, safe implementation of the calorie restriction (CR) pattern in geriatric adults may not be possible. Because anorexia and/or malnutrition tendencies are frequently observed in these individuals [29]. In this context, long-term calorie restriction may not be an appropriate anti-aging nutritional model for geriatric adults.

Considering this situation, intermittent fasting (IF) has received remarkable attention as an alternative dietary pattern as a more feasible and effective dietary regimen than continuous calorie restriction, which carries the risk of malnutrition [30]. Some individuals, especially older adults, can more easily maintain IF (time-restricted eating) methods than continuous calorie restriction and single-food-group-based eating patterns. For example, in a study conducted by Conley and colleagues in 2018, participants aged 67 and over successfully implemented this diet regimen that lasted 6 months [31].

4. Intermittent fasting, metabolic effects and autophagy

The effects of the intermittent fasting model on human physiology and aging mechanisms have attracted much attention from scientists and the media and have been the subject of many studies. Intermittent fasting (IF), which is an easier model to implement than the classical calorie restriction model, is a model that severely restricts calorie intake during part of the day and allows calorie-free nutrition during the remaining time of the day (eating window). Taking into account the person's age, health status, metabolism and chronic diseases, personalized meal models can be created and fasting hours can start from 12 hours and can be extended up to 14-16-20 hours (time-restricted IF). Although time-restricted IF is the most common and applicable form of IF, it can be divided into four main headings: alternate-day fasting, alternate-day modified fasting and 5:2 IF.

Alternate-day fasting (ADF); is a type of IF based on alternating days of free calorie intake with days of complete prohibition of calorie intake. Considering the difficulties experienced by participants who do not comply with this model, the IF model that allows the consumption of some calories (310–380 kcal) during fasting periods is called alternate-day modified fasting (ADMF) [32]. Another type of IF, the 5:2 IF model, is a model in which eating is allowed for 5 days a week, while severe energy restriction or complete fasting is performed on the other 2 days. Since there are insufficient studies proving the reliability of long-term fasting in geriatric age groups, the model that can be safely sustained compared to these three models is the time-restrictive IF model [31].

Time-restricted feeding (TRF) involves restricting daily calorie intake to a period of time, usually between 12 and 4 hours. This protocol involves fasting periods of 12–20 hours. Because TRF involves eating meals mostly during the day and fasting at night, it is more effective at regulating circadian rhythms than other types of intermittent fasting (IF).

The effects of intermittent fasting, which has been the subject of many studies due to its proven effects on human physiology and aging, on human metabolism can be explained as follows; One of the most important mechanisms of intermittent fasting (IF) is to change the metabolic phases of organisms during fasting periods, improving metabolic conditions and prolonging the duration of the healthy state. It does this by triggering defense mechanisms against oxidative and metabolic stress through autophagy and by suppressing inflammation. This effect of IF is similar to the metabolic effect provided by aerobic exercise [33]. In glucose and amino acid deprivation, AMP-activated protein kinase (AMPK) activity is stimulated and the mTOR signaling pathway is inhibited. These changes induce autophagy and oxidative defense mechanisms by inhibiting FOXO gene transcription [34]. In addition, body rejuvenation and repair are activated.

The Nobel Prize in Physiology or Medicine in 2016 was awarded to Yoshinori Ohsumi in 1990 for being the first scientist to explain the mechanism of autophagy at the morphological and molecular level. Autophagy breaks down macromolecules and damaged organelles, increases mitochondrial efficiency and supports the survival of cells under constant stress [35]. While the basal autophagy rate of normal cells continues at low levels under physiological conditions, a high level of basal autophagy mechanism operates in some tumoral cells, supporting the pro-survival role of autophagy in cancer [36]. Autophagy also acts as a decelerator in the metastasis process by intervening in the epithelial-mesenchymal transition (EMT) component to slow down the spread of tumoral cells. The fact that fasting periods are one of the most important triggers of autophagy and protect against oxidative damage by activating antioxidant defenses [37] has enabled the IF nutritional model to take place in the treatment of cancer patients.

It is noteworthy that the IF nutritional model can prevent the precursors of aging by regulating the basic components of metabolic syndrome, insulin resistance and B-oxidation of lipids. When the physiology of diabetes is examined in the studies conducted, it is shown that lipid metabolism disorders develop diabetes by disrupting glucose metabolism through insulin resistance and can cause permanent insulin resistance [38].

A clinical study in patients with type 2 diabetes (T2DM) showed that 12 months of intermittent fasting (IF) resulted in significant reductions in body weight, glycated hemoglobin levels (HgbA1c), fasting glucose and insulin levels [39]. In a different clinical study, it was proven that time-restricted IF significantly reduced insulin levels and improved insulin sensitivity and pancreatic β-cell sensitivity. It was shown that this decrease in insulin was more pronounced with IF compared to the calorie restriction (CR) model [40].

When geriatric metabolism is examined, chronic inflammation, which is one of the basic mechanisms of aging, is associated with insulin resistance, high CRP (C-reactive protein), decreased adiponectin (Adiponectin is an adipokine derived from fat tissue with anti-atherosclerotic and anti-inflammatory properties), low-density lipoprotein and the development of coronary artery disease and atherosclerosis [41]. When controlled and non-aggressive fasting-eating periods are included in the diet of cardiac patients, it has been observed that the basic pathology, insulin resistance, is broken, hepatic fatty acid oxidation is increased and triglyceride accumulation is reduced. This, in turn, has been found to reduce hepatic very low density lipoprotein (VLDL) production and plasma VLDL levels. And it has been observed that this significantly improves cardiac metabolism by improving the lipid profile [42].

If we examine the effect of the IF model on fat metabolism more closely, it is aimed to prevent excessive fat storage in geriatric individuals with aging and to have the potential to treat lipid-related diseases. Although obesity is not a very common problem in the elderly, studies show that the geriatric population is at risk for central obesity in the future. According to National Health Insurance Service study data, the rate of obesity in adults aged 71–79 was 31% in 2006, increasing to 37% in 2015. In individuals aged 80 and over, the rate of obesity was found to have increased from 22% in 2006 to 28% in 2015 [43]. Geriatric individuals are largely protected from the typical central obesity and metabolic syndrome of aging by living an active life and preventing excessive fat gain through a consistent diet.

Another metabolic process that is inevitable in the aging process of geriatric individuals is the decline in neurocognitive activities. Although it is not possible to eliminate this decline, clinical studies have proven that IF has the potential to slow down this process. These studies have revealed that IF can support synaptic plasticity, neuroprotection processes and neurogenesis, especially by increasing the expression of brain-derived neurotrophic factor (BDNF) [44]. Another IF feeding study found that the mechanisms of recovery were increased neuronal resistance to excitotoxic stress, prevention of learning disorders caused by hippocampal cell death and promotion of neurogenesis [45]. These findings shed light on the potential therapeutic effects of IF in preventing neurodegenerative diseases and slowing down age-related cognitive decline.

The effects and mechanisms of intermittent fasting (IF) on metabolic and physiological processes have been investigated, as proven by many clinical studies conducted on young, adult and geriatric individuals. Studies show that the IF nutritional model has significant healing potential in terms of its effects on glucose-insulin metabolism, fatty acid metabolism, cellular immunity and inflammation, cardiac and neurocognitive health, and is a preferred nutritional model for a long and healthy life. The Time-Restricted IF diet, which is more sustainable than other single-type food sources or excessive calorie and time-restricted nutrition models, is the diet model that has the most successful patient compliance and is most suitable for the circadian rhythm. For this reason, studies have shown that the IF nutrition model, which is started at a young and adult age and continued under control in the geriatric period, can be a beneficial nonpharmacological intervention for long life. This nutritional model, which may contribute to the slowing down of aging physiology, has points and patient groups that need to be taken into consideration, as in every nutritional and therapeutic treatment. An individual-specific approach and planning is an indisputable necessity in all pharmacological or nonpharmacological therapeutic approaches.

The IF nutritional model should not be applied to diabetic patients who are using glucose-lowering medications, especially those with uncontrolled and irregular fasting, and those with kidney parameters that may lead to hypoglycemia or kidney damage [46]. However, with patient education and ensuring that the drug dosage does not cause hypoglycemia or that the IF diet is controlled and the eating window is not too short in prediabetic patients who are being followed without medication, it can be applied [47]. This model should also not be applied to critically ill or cachectic elderly individuals, sick neonates, infants and young children. Clinical studies including this critical group have shown that, although it does not cause hypoglycemia in children under 1 year of age, it slightly increases ketosis [48]. In addition, a clinical IF study with drugs has shown that it increases the cardiotoxic side effects of doxorubicin in animal models that are continuously subjected to a time-restricted feeding model, which should be considered first in patients receiving chemotherapy [49].

5. Conclusion

In this study, physiological and pathophysiological mechanisms of aging were discussed and the importance of nonpharmacological approaches that will support healthy and long life was emphasized once again. It was explained that with increasing life expectancy, aging, which is an inevitable end, can become a manageable clinical picture with correct lifestyle interventions. Intermittent fasting, which has been proven by clinical studies to be one of the most suitable nutritional models for circadian rhythm and has the potential to improve age-related metabolic changes, has been highlighted. This nutritional model, which should be planned specifically for each individual, considering the individual's metabolic and comorbid conditions in all age groups, will be a major and critical step in the aging process, with the aim of maintaining sustainable geriatric health.

Author details

Hilal Demirci
Department of Family Medicine, School of Medicine, Kafkas University, Kars, Turkey

*Address all correspondence to: dr.demircihilal@gmail.com

References

[1] López-Otín C, Blasco MA, Partridge L, Serrano M, Kroemer G. The hallmarks of aging. Cell. 2013;**153**(6):1192-1219

[2] Kirkwood TBL. Understanding the odd science of aging. Cell. 2005;**120**(4):435-449

[3] United Nations, Population Division. World Population Prospects 2017 Revision: Key Findings and Advanced Tables (Report No. ST/ESA/SER.A/416). New York, NY: United Nations Department of Economic and Social Affairs, Population Division; 2017. Available from: https://population.un.org/wpp/Publications/Files/WPP2017_KeyFindings.pdf

[4] United Nations, Department of Economic and Social Affairs, Population Division. The Extent and Rate of Population Aging (World Population Ageing 1950-2050, Part II). New York: United Nations; 2011. Available from: http://www.un.org/esa/population/publications/worldageing19502050/pdf/80chapterii.pdf

[5] Salmon AB, Richardson A, Pérez VI. Update on the oxidative stress theory of aging: Does oxidative stress play a role in aging or healthy aging? Free Radical Biology & Medicine. 2010;**48**:642-655

[6] Haigis MC, Yankner BA. Aging stress response. Molecular Cell. 2010;**40**:333-344

[7] Hazen R. Strategic Nutrition for Healthy Aging [Technical Article]. Chicago, Illinois, USA: Fortitech Premixes; Mar 2014. Available from: http://www.fortitechpremixes.com/wp-content/uploads/2014/02/Healthy_Aging_EN.pdf

[8] Rattan SIS, Sejersen H, Fernandes RA, Luo W. Stress-mediated hormetic modulation of aging, wound healing, and angiogenesis in human cells. Annals of the New York Academy of Sciences. 2007;**1119**:112-121

[9] Alberti KGMM, Eckel RH, Grundy SM, Zimmet PZ, Cleeman JI, Donato KA, et al. Harmonization of the metabolic syndrome: Joint interim statement of the task force on epidemiology and prevention of the International Diabetes Federation; National Heart, Lung, and Blood Institute; American Heart Association; World Heart Federation; International Atherosclerosis Society; and International Association for the Study of Obesity. Circulation. 2009;**120**:1639-1646

[10] Cano-Ibáñez N, Gea A, Martínez-González MA, Salas-Salvadó J, Corella D, Zomeño MD, et al. Dietary diversity and nutrient adequacy in an elderly Spanish population with metabolic syndrome in the PREDIMED-plus study: A cross-sectional analysis. Nutrients. 2019;**11**:958

[11] Julibert A, Bibiloni MDM, Mateos D, Angullo E, Tur JA. Dietary fat intake and metabolic syndrome in older adults. Nutrients. 2019;**11**(8):1901. DOI: 10.3390/nu11081901

[12] Storniolo CE, Sacanella I, Mitjavila MT, Lamuela-Raventós RM, Moreno JJ. Bioactive compounds of cooked tomato sauce regulate oxidative stress and arachidonic acid cascade induced by oxidized LDL in macrophage cultures. Nutrients. 2019;**11**(8):1880. DOI: 10.3390/nu11081880

[13] Osti V, Bertozzi B, Fontana L. Health benefits of the Mediterranean diet:

Metabolic and molecular mechanisms. The Journals of Gerontology. Series A, Biological Sciences and Medical Sciences. 2018;**73**:317-327

[14] Chiva-Blanch G, Badimon L. Effects of polyphenol intake on metabolic syndrome: Current evidence from human experiments. Oxidative Medicine and Cellular Longevity. 2017;**2017**:5812401

[15] Finicelli M, Squillaro T, Di Cristo F, Di Salle A, Kavun MAB, Galderisi U, et al. Metabolic syndrome, Mediterranean diet, and polyphenols: Evidence and perspectives. Journal of Cellular Physiology. 2019;**234**:5806-5827

[16] Soltani S, Jayedi A, Shab-Bidar S, Becerra-Tomás N, Salas-Salvadó J. Association of Mediterranean diet adherence with all-cause mortality: A systematic review and dose-response meta-analysis of prospective cohort studies. Advances in Nutrition. 2019;**10**:1028-1040

[17] Martínez-González MA, Gea A, Ruiz-Canela M. Mediterranean diet and cardiovascular health. Circulation Research. 2019;**124**(5):779-798. DOI: 10.1161/CIRCRESAHA.118.313348

[18] Ge L, Sadeghirad B, Ball GDC, Da Costa BR, Hitchcock CL, Svendrovski A, et al. Comparison of dietary macronutrient patterns of 14 popular named dietary programs for the reduction of weight and cardiovascular risk factors in adults: A systematic review and network meta-analysis of randomized trials. BMJ. 2020;**369**:m696

[19] U.S. Department of Health and Human Services. Dash Diet. In: Handbook of Disease Burdens and Quality of Life Measures. Bethesda, MD, USA: National Institutes of Health, National Heart, Lung, and Blood Institute; 2010

[20] Phillips CM, Harrington JM, Perry IJ. Association between diet quality determined by the DASH score and biomarkers of cardiometabolic health: A cross-sectional analysis in adults. Clinical Nutrition. 2019;**38**:1619-1629

[21] Mozaffarian D. Diet and policy priorities for cardiovascular disease, diabetes, and obesity: A comprehensive review. Circulation. 2016;**133**:186-226

[22] Paoli A, Rubini A, Volek JS, Grimaldi KA. Beyond weight loss: A review of therapeutic uses of very-low-carbohydrate (ketogenic) diets. European Journal of Clinical Nutrition. 2013;**67**:790-797

[23] Jensen MD, Ryan DH, Apovian CM, Ard JD, Comuzzie AG, Donato KA, et al. 2013 AHA/ACC/TOS guideline for the management of overweight and obesity in adults: A report of the American College of Cardiology/American Heart Association Practice Guidelines Task Force and the Obesity Society. Circulation. 2014;**129**(Supplement_3):S102-S138. DOI: 10.1161/01.cir.0000437739.71477.ee

[24] Choi HR, Kim J, Lim H, Park YK. Two-week supplementation with a specially modified ketogenic nutritional beverage preserves lean body mass and improves blood lipid profile in obese adults: A randomized clinical trial. Nutrients. 2018;**10**(12):1895. DOI: 10.3390/nu10121895

[25] Uusitupa M, Hermansen K, Savolainen MJ, Schwab U, Kolehmainen M, Brader L, et al. Effects of an isocaloric healthy Scandinavian diet on insulin sensitivity, lipid profile, and markers of inflammation in the metabolic syndrome - A randomized trial (SYSDIET). Journal of Internal Medicine. 2013;**274**:51-67

[26] Bojang KP, Manchana V, et al. Nutrition and healthy aging: A review. Current Nutrition Reports. 2023;**12**(3):369-375. DOI: 10.1007/s13668-023-00473-0

[27] Redman LM, Ravussin E. Caloric restriction in humans: Physiological, psychological, and behavioral effects. Antioxidants and Redox Signaling. 2011;**14**(2):275-287. DOI: 10.1089/ars.2010.3253

[28] Ravussin E, Redman LM, Rochon J, Das SK, Fontana L, Kraus WE, et al. A 2-year randomized controlled trial of calorie restriction in humans: Feasibility and effects on predictors of healthy lifespan and longevity. Journals of Gerontology: Series A, Biological Sciences and Medical Sciences. 2015;**70**(9):1097-1104. DOI: 10.1093/gerona/glv057

[29] Wysokinski A, Sobow T, Kloszewska I, Kostka T. Mechanisms of anorexia in aging. Age (Dordrecht, Netherlands). 2015;**37**(4):9822

[30] Cioffi I, Evangelista A, Ponzo V, Ciccone G, Soldati L, Santarpia L, et al. Effect of intermittent and continuous energy restriction on weight loss and cardiometabolic outcomes: A systematic review and meta-analysis of randomized controlled trials. Journal of Translational Medicine. 2018;**16**(1):370

[31] Conley M, Le Fevre L, Haywood C, Proietto J. Is two days per week of intermittent energy restriction a feasible weight loss approach in obese men? A Randomized Pilot Study. 2018;**75**(1):64-73

[32] Johnson JB, Summer W, Cutler RG, Martin B, Hyun DH, Dixit VD, et al. Alternate-day calorie restriction improves clinical findings and reduces oxidative stress and inflammatory markers in overweight adults with moderate asthma. Free Radical Biology and Medicine. 2007;**42**(5):665-674. DOI: 10.1016/j.freeradbiomed.2006.12.005

[33] Schübel R, Nattenmüller J, Sookthai D, Nonnenmacher T, Graf ME, Riedl L, et al. Effects of intermittent and continuous calorie restriction on body weight and metabolism during 50 weeks: Randomized controlled trial. The American Journal of Clinical Nutrition. 2018;**108**:932-946

[34] Green CL, Lamming DW, Fontana L. Molecular mechanisms of dietary restriction that promote health and longevity. Nature Reviews. Molecular Cell Biology. 2022;**23**:55-74

[35] Kroemer G, Marião G, Levine B. Autophagy and the integrated stress response. Molecular Cell. 2010;**40**(2):279-294

[36] White E. The role of autophagy in cancer. The Journal of Clinical Investigation. 2015;**125**(1):42-46

[37] Castello L, Froio T, Maina M, Cavallini G, Biasi F, Leonarduzzi G. Alternate-day fasting protects rat heart against age-related inflammation and fibrosis by inhibiting oxidative damage and NF-kB activation. Free Radical Biology & Medicine. 2010;**48**:47-54

[38] Lambert JE. Parks, EJ postprandial metabolism of food triglycerides in humans. Biochimica et Biophysica Acta. 2012;**1821**:722-727

[39] Carter S, Clifton PM, Keogh JB. Effect of intermittent and continuous energy-restricted diets on glycemic control in patients with type 2 diabetes: A randomized non-inferiority study. JAMA Network Open. 2018;**1**:e180756

[40] Cioffi I, Evangelista A, Ponzo V, Ciccone G, Soldati L, Santarpia L, et al. Effect of intermittent and continuous energy restriction on weight loss and cardiometabolic outcomes: A systematic review and meta-analysis of randomized controlled trials. Journal of Translational Medicine. 2018;**16**:371

[41] Shulman GI. Ectopic fat in insulin resistance, dyslipidemia, and cardiometabolic disease. The New England Journal of Medicine. 2014;**371**:2236-2239

[42] Wang YX. PPARs: Various regulators in energy metabolism and metabolic diseases. Cell Research. 2010;**20**:123-3711

[43] Seo MH, Kim YH, Han K, Jung JH, Park YG, Lee SS, et al. Prevalence of obesity and incidence of obesity-related comorbidities in Koreans according to national health insurance service health check-up data 2006-2015. Journal of Obesity & Metabolic Syndrome. 2018;**27**:45-53

[44] Kaptan Z, Akgün-Dar K, Kapucu A, Dedeakayogulları H, Batu S, Üzüm G. Long-term effects of a low-calorie diet during adolescence on spatial learning and memory in female rats; BDNF levels in the hippocampus and prefrontal cortex, NeuN expression, and cell proliferation in the dentate gyrus. Brain Research. 2015;**1618**:194-204. DOI: 10.1016/j.brainres.2015.05.041

[45] Qiu G, Spangler EL, Wan R, Miller M, Mattson MP, So KF, et al. Neuroprotection conferred by dietary restriction is further enhanced by reducing glucocorticoids in rats. Aging Cell. 2012;**11**(4):733-740. DOI: 10.1111/j.1474-9726.2012.00835.x

[46] Al-Ozairi E, El Samad A, Al Kandari J, Aldibbiat AM. Intermittent fasting can be performed safely in individuals with type 1 diabetes mellitus undergoing structured training and advanced glucose monitoring. Frontiers Endocrinology (Lausanne). 2019;**10**:850

[47] Corley BT, Carroll RW, Hall RM, Weatherall M, Parry-Strong A, Krebs JD. Intermittent fasting and risk of hypoglycemia in type 2 diabetes mellitus: A randomized controlled trial. Diabetic Medicine. 2018;**35**(5):587-595

[48] Veldscholte K, Cramer ABG, de Jonge RCJ, Rizopoulos D, Joosten KFM, Verbruggen S. Comparison of overnight fasting with intermittent feeding and 24-h feeding in critically ill neonates, infants, and children: An open-label, single-center, randomized controlled trial. Clinical Nutrition. 2023;**42**(9):1568-1581

[49] Ozcan M, Guo Z, Valenzuela Ripoll C, Diab A, Picataggi A, Rawnsley D, et al. Continuous alternate-day fasting potentiates doxorubicin cardiotoxicity. Cell Metabolism. 2023;**35**(6):927-943

Chapter 9

The Contribution of AI to Our Thinking of the Intersection of Longevity and Food Habits

Howard R. Moskowitz and Sharon Wingert

Abstract

With AI acting as both a research assistant and co-author, this paper shows how one can rapidly create a knowledge base about the intersection of AI and food/nutrition as they drive longevity. The paper treats the topic through seven distinct foci, all involving generative AI. Focus 1 simulates how the general population would feel when they learn that nutritional science is being integrated into AI to provide actionable recommendations. Focus 2 simulates how nutrition professionals react when they learn how nutritional information is combined with AI. Focus 3 uses Mind Genomics thinking to simulate the four mind-sets in each of two groups (general population professionals and nutritional professionals) as these minds consider the role of AI in nutrition. Focus 4 simulates viewpoints regarding incorporating AI in the nutrition-longevity link. Focus 5 uses AI-based critical thinking to identify themes and perspectives. In Focus 6, AI presents AI-suggested process innovations for nutrition to increase longevity. Focus 7 uses AI to pose relevant questions and generate answers. The paper shows the power of AI as a partner in helping to develop insights prior to empirical research.

Keywords: AI in nutrition, AI in research, generative AI applications, longevity and diet, mind genomics thinking, personalized nutrition strategies

1. Introduction

AI reveals intricate links among longevity, dietary habits, nutrition, and our perceptions of food. Employing AI to analyze vast amounts of data uncovers complex patterns and connections and may provide deep insights into how our dietary decisions impact health and longevity [1–4].

Studying the diets of individuals who have thrived throughout history may reveal foods and nutrients associated with increased longevity. Additionally, AI indicates how our perspectives on food and eating habits affect our lifespan. By analyzing social media posts, surveys, and diverse data sources, AI reveals common attitudes and behaviors surrounding food that may impact longevity, either favorably or unfavorably, respectively [5–8].

AI is useful in developing personalized nutrition plans that take into account individual factors such as genetics, lifestyle, and health conditions. By analyzing an

IntechOpen

individual's eating habits and nutritional needs, as well as their views on food, AI provides tailored recommendations designed to enhance longevity and overall well-being. Furthermore, AI dispels myths and misconceptions surrounding nutrition and longevity by providing clear, evidence-based guidance and insights.

Considering the previous points, we now explore various connections between the capabilities of modern AI and the prospects for longevity. This paper employs AI as its research and writing assistant. This paper aims to develop a method for exploring the significant connection between longevity and nutritional attitudes and behaviors, relying entirely on AI to conduct the analysis. Should the effort prove successful, society will gain a new instrument to address its challenges with a focus on knowledge [9–11].

2. Focus 1: AI simulates how the general population would feel when they learn that nutritional science is being integrated into AI to provide actionable recommendations

In a rapidly evolving world shaped by technological advancements, the fusion of nutritional science with artificial intelligence emerges as a transformative force, poised to redefine our approach to health and wellness. With AI configured to deliver actionable insights rooted in nutritional science, individuals can generate tailored information, enabling them to make informed choices about their diets and overall well-being. This integration can enable individuals to seize control of their well-being, fostering positive changes that enhance their quality of life. AI provides personalized recommendations that consider individual needs and preferences, resulting in more effective and sustainable outcomes.

The world will likely respond to this innovation with a blend of excitement, curiosity, and skepticism as individuals navigate the implications of depending on technology for nutritional guidance. Some individuals may welcome the concept of a virtual nutritionist readily available, while others might question the precision and trustworthiness of AI-generated advice. Yet, the prevailing sentiment is expected to be one of intrigue and captivation as society embraces this emerging realm of health technology. **Table 1** shows how AI synthesizes the "world of AI + nutrition" into a capsule discussion of the response to AI [12, 13].

AI Instructed to Write a Composition Focusing on How the World Feels About Knowing that a Lot of Its Nutritional Science is Being Integrated into AI to Provide Actionable Recommendations
1. Nutritional science is essential for grasping the impact of food on our bodies and overall well-being. With the progression of technology, AI is progressively employed to sift through extensive data, delivering tailored recommendations that cater to an individual's distinct requirements. Integrating nutritional science with AI allows us to harness the latest research and findings, crafting precise and dependable recommendations for those looking to enhance their diet and health. This integration enables AI to decode intricate nutritional data and deliver actionable insights instantly, empowering users to make well-informed dietary decisions.
2. A major advantage of merging nutritional science with AI lies in its capacity to deliver tailored recommendations that align with a person's unique health objectives, dietary choices, and lifestyle considerations. AI algorithms sift through diverse data, such as personal biometric information, dietary habits, and medical backgrounds, crafting personalized recommendations that resonate with each individual. Leveraging AI to merge nutritional science, enabling individuals to seize control of their health and well-being through informed dietary choices. This integration transforms our approach to nutrition, offering insights that were once hard to access or required significant time to uncover.

3. Additionally, incorporating nutritional science into AI connects scientific research with real-world applications. It achieves this by transforming intricate data into clear, actionable recommendations that are straightforward to grasp and apply. AI algorithms scrutinize nutritional data, revealing trends and patterns that highlight the connections between diet and health outcomes, empowering individuals to make informed decisions about their food choices. This integration empowers healthcare professionals to deliver tailored dietary advice to their patients, resulting in enhanced health outcomes and an improved quality of life.
4. Integrating nutritional science with AI tackles the rising issue of food insecurity by offering personalized suggestions for those who struggle to access healthy foods. AI algorithms assess food availability, dietary preferences, and cultural norms, providing tailored suggestions that are practical and sustainable for individuals across various socioeconomic backgrounds. This integration highlights food deserts and regions with restricted access to healthy foods, allowing policymakers to create focused interventions that tackle these inequalities and enhance nutrition outcomes in underserved communities.
5. Integrating nutritional science with AI facilitates ongoing monitoring and feedback on dietary habits, empowering individuals to track their progress and make real-time adjustments. AI algorithms assess food intake, physical activity, sleep patterns, and various lifestyle factors, crafting personalized recommendations that cater to everyone's distinct needs and preferences. This integration aids individuals in recognizing harmful patterns and behaviors. Integrating AI with nutritional science fosters a proactive and preventive healthcare strategy.
6. Integrating nutritional science into AI tackles the rising issue of chronic diseases and health conditions associated with unhealthy eating habits. AI algorithms sift through extensive data from diverse populations to uncover risk factors and trends linked to diet-related diseases like diabetes, heart disease, and obesity. Policymakers and healthcare providers create focused strategies that encourage healthier eating habits, effectively preventing the emergence of these conditions. The integration offers tailored suggestions that enhance their treatment plans.
7. Evidence-based recommendations are customized to fit an individual's specific needs and preferences. AI algorithms examine dietary patterns, cooking habits, food preferences, and cultural traditions to provide relevant and practical personalization. This integration empowers educators and nutrition professionals to create more focused and effective interventions.
8. AI algorithms examine data related to food sourcing, production techniques, and transportation trends to evaluate the environmental impact of various foods, providing recommendations that align with sustainability principles. This integration reveals the links between our dietary choices and significant global challenges like climate change, deforestation, and biodiversity loss, enabling individuals to make informed decisions that foster a healthier planet for generations to come.

Table 1.
The AI synthesis of how the world feels about knowing that a lot of nutritional science is being integrated into AI to provide actionable recommendations.

3. Focus 2: AI simulates how nutrition professionals react when they learn how nutrition information is being combined with AI

By understanding the perspectives and concerns of nutrition professionals towards AI as shown in **Table 2**, we anticipate potential challenges and opportunities that may arise. This information can help guide the development and implementation of AI technology in the field of nutrition, ensuring that it is beneficial and accepted by professionals in the industry. Further, we may forestall and even nullify any attitude problems emerging when professionals end up feeling threatened that technology will replace them [14–17].

AI Simulates How Nutrition Professionals React When They Learn How Nutrition Information is Being Combined with AI
1. Experts in nutrition and healthcare might respond differently to the application of AI in suggesting dietary behaviors aimed at promoting longevity. Their responses can be shaped by numerous factors, such as personal beliefs and values, professional training and experience, and their attitudes towards technology and innovation. Some professionals may eagerly anticipate AI's potential to enhance health outcomes and optimize their practices, whereas others may harbor concerns regarding the ethical implications and limitations of AI in healthcare.
2. Many professionals see AI as a powerful tool that tailors recommendations for their clients, leading to better health outcomes. They might value AI's capacity to sift through vast data sets, delivering personalized, evidence-based recommendations that cater to unique needs and preferences. These professionals are likely thrilled by the prospect of AI elevating their practice, streamlining their work, and boosting effectiveness.
3. Certain professionals might express reservations regarding the application of AI providing nutrition advice aimed at enhancing longevity. Concerns arise regarding the accuracy and reliability of AI algorithms, particularly in relation to intricate and subtle subjects such as nutrition. These professionals might worry that AI suggestions could lack specificity, resulting in less-than-ideal results for their clients. Concerns arise regarding AI's potential to supplant human expertise and empathy in healthcare, risking the loss of the personal touch and individualized care that clients deeply appreciate.
4. Some professionals express ethical concerns regarding the application of AI providing nutrition recommendations aimed at enhancing longevity. Concerns may arise regarding data privacy and security, alongside the risk of bias and discrimination inherent in AI algorithms. These professionals might be wary of relying on AI for sensitive personal information and decisions concerning health and well-being. They might experience a duty to maintain ethical standards and safeguard their clients' interests, even amidst the rise of technological advancements.
5. Professionals who hold an optimistic perspective on AI recognize its potential advantages in providing nutrition recommendations aimed at enhancing longevity. They might welcome innovative technologies and methods that could enhance health outcomes and elevate the quality of life for their clients. These professionals might wonder how AI can elevate their practice and keep them updated on the newest research and optimal strategies in nutrition and longevity. They are keen to delve into the potential of AI, weaving it into their work to enrich their expertise and elevate the care they offer to their clients.
6. Some professionals, taking a more cautious stance on AI, may choose to depend on their own expertise and experience when offering nutrition advice for longevity. They likely appreciate the human aspect of healthcare, viewing personalized care and empathy as vital elements of successful treatment. These professionals might doubt AI's capacity to effectively evaluate and cater to the distinct needs and preferences of each client. They might choose a more engaged method for nutrition counseling, valuing personal interaction and teamwork with their clients rather than relying on automated AI-generated suggestions.

Table 2.
AI simulations showing how nutrition professionals react when they learn how nutrition information is being combined with AI.

4. Focus 3: Using mind genomics thinking to simulate the four mind-sets in each of the two groups (general population professionals and nutritional professionals)

Mind Genomics reveals concealed preferences and biases that shape professionals' interpretation and application of nutritional information. A deeper understanding allows us to pinpoint areas of agreement and conflict within the field, paving the way for more informed and effective strategies to promote healthy eating habits. Combining AI technology with insights from Mind Genomics thinking produces a deeper and more detailed understanding of nutrition, benefiting both professionals and consumers alike. This fusion of AI and Mind Genomics could transform our approach to nutrition and health, paving the way for more effective strategies that enhance overall well-being. **Table 3** shows how AI creates two different groups of four mind-sets each. The first group comprises the thinking of ordinary people about AI and nutrition while the second group is for the thinking of professionals about AI and nutrition [18–22].

GROUP 1: FOUR MIND-SETS OF THE "GENERAL PROFESSIONAL" REGARDING AI IN NUTRITION

NAME: Traditionalists
BELIEVE: Traditionalists believe that AI helps analyze data and make recommendations for nutrition-driven longevity. They see AI as a tool to gather and interpret large amounts of data more efficiently than humans could on their own. Traditionalists also believe that AI algorithms identify patterns and correlations that may not be immediately apparent to human researchers, leading to more personalized recommendations for individuals.

COUNTERING CRITICS: Traditionalists may defend themselves against critics by highlighting the potential benefits of AI in improving overall health outcomes and quality of life. They may point to studies that have shown AI to be an effective tool in predicting and preventing chronic diseases. Traditionalists may also emphasize the role of human oversight in ensuring that AI recommendations are accurate and evidence based.

EVOLVING TO 2030: In the year 2030, Traditionalists may evolve their thinking by integrating more advanced AI technologies, such as machine learning and deep learning, into their analysis and recommendations. They may also work towards incorporating real-time data and feedback from wearable devices and smart technology into their algorithms, allowing for even more personalized and precise nutrition recommendations.

NAME: Skeptics
BELIEVE: Skeptics are cautious about using AI to guide thinking about nutrition-driven longevity. They believe that AI algorithms may not always be reliable or accurate in their recommendations, especially when they do not consider individual differences and nuances. Skeptics also worry about the potential for bias in AI algorithms, which could lead to misleading or harmful recommendations.

COUNTERING CRITICS: Skeptics may defend themselves against critics by emphasizing the importance of human judgment and critical thinking in interpreting AI recommendations. They may also point to cases where AI algorithms have made errors or incorrect predictions, highlighting the limitations of relying solely on AI for nutrition guidance. Skeptics may call for more transparency and oversight in the development and implementation of AI technology in the field of nutrition.

EVOLVING TO 2030: In the year 2030, Skeptics may evolve their thinking by advocating for more rigorous validation and testing of AI algorithms used in nutrition recommendations. They may also push for greater collaboration between AI researchers and nutrition experts to ensure that AI algorithms consider the latest scientific evidence and best practices in nutrition. Skeptics may work towards developing more robust safeguards and checks to prevent bias and errors in AI recommendations.
NAME: Optimists

BELIEVE: Optimists are enthusiastic about the potential of AI to revolutionize nutrition-driven longevity. They believe that AI has the capacity to analyze vast amounts of data, from genetics to lifestyle factors, and provide personalized recommendations that significantly improve individual health outcomes. Optimists see AI as a powerful tool that help individuals make more informed decisions about their diets and lifestyles, leading to longer and healthier lives.

COUNTERING CRITICS: Optimists may defend themselves against critics by highlighting the success stories of AI in improving health outcomes and extending lifespans. They may point to studies that have shown AI to be more accurate and reliable than traditional methods in predicting and preventing diseases. Optimists may also emphasize the need for continuous research and development to further enhance the capabilities of AI in the field of nutrition.

EVOLVING TO 2030: In the year 2030, Optimists may continue to advocate for the integration of advanced AI technologies, such as artificial neural networks and natural language processing, into nutrition analysis and recommendations. They may also focus on using AI to promote behavioral changes and adherence to healthy eating habits, through interactive apps and virtual assistants. Optimists may work towards increasing access to AI-powered nutrition tools for a wider population, through smartphone apps and online platforms.

NAME: Ethicists
BELIEVE: Ethicists are concerned about the potential ethical implications of using AI to guide thinking about nutrition-driven longevity. They believe that AI algorithms may perpetuate biases and inequalities in healthcare, by favoring certain populations or promoting certain dietary trends. Ethicists also worry about the privacy and security risks associated with collecting and analyzing personal health data using AI technologies.

COUNTERING CRITICS: Ethicists may defend themselves against critics by emphasizing the importance of ethical guidelines and principles in the development and implementation of AI in nutrition recommendations. They may call for greater transparency and accountability in how AI algorithms are trained and deployed, to ensure fairness and equity in the recommendations provided. Ethicists may also advocate for the active involvement of diverse stakeholder groups, such as patient advocates and community organizations, in shaping the ethical framework for AI-driven nutrition interventions.

EVOLVING TO 2030: In the year 2030, Ethicists may evolve their thinking by pushing for the establishment of clear regulations and standards governing the use of AI in nutrition recommendations. They may also work towards promoting education and awareness among the public about the ethical considerations related to AI in healthcare. Ethicists may advocate for the development of AI technologies that prioritize privacy and data security, while still delivering accurate and personalized nutrition guidance.

GROUP 2: FOUR MIND-SETS OF THE "NUTRITION-INVOLVED PROFESSIONAL" REGARDING AI IN NUTRITION
NAME: Data Scientists
BELIEVE: Data Scientists believe that AI provides personalized nutrition recommendations based on extensive data analysis, leading to improved health outcomes and increased longevity. AI algorithms analyze individual biological markers, dietary preferences, and lifestyle habits to tailor nutrition plans for optimal wellness. They also recognize the potential for AI to revolutionize the healthcare industry by providing real-time monitoring and feedback on an individual's nutritional needs.

COUNTERING CRITICS: Data Scientists defend their use of AI in nutrition-driven longevity by highlighting the rigor and accuracy of data analysis techniques used in their algorithms. They argue that data-driven recommendations are more precise and effective than traditional one-size-fits-all approaches. Additionally, they emphasize the importance of ongoing validation and refinement of AI models to ensure reliability and safety.

EVOLVING TO 2030: In the year 2030, Data Scientists are likely to further refine their AI algorithms to incorporate a wider range of data sources, including genetic information, microbiome analysis, and environmental factors. They may also explore the integration of AI technology with wearable devices for continuous monitoring and feedback on nutritional choices. Data Scientists could lead the development of AI-powered personalized nutrition platforms that are widely accessible and affordable for individuals seeking to optimize their longevity.

NAME: Medical Professionals
BELIEVE: Medical Professionals believe that AI enhances the practice of personalized medicine by providing evidence-based nutritional recommendations tailored to an individual's unique health profile. They understand the significance of nutrition in preventing chronic diseases and promoting longevity, and view AI as a valuable tool in optimizing patient outcomes. Medical Professionals value the ability of AI algorithms to process large datasets and meta-analyses to generate actionable insights for clinical practice.

COUNTERING CRITICS: Medical Professionals defend their reliance on AI by highlighting the extensive training and expertise required to interpret and apply nutritional guidelines effectively. They argue that AI complements rather than replaces human expertise, facilitating more efficient and data-driven decision-making in patient care. Medical Professionals emphasize the importance of continual education and professional development to stay abreast of technological advancements in healthcare.

EVOLVING TO 2030: By 2030, Medical Professionals may further integrate AI technologies into clinical practice to support patient engagement and compliance with personalized nutrition plans. They could collaborate with data scientists and nutritionists to develop comprehensive digital health platforms that combine medical knowledge with AI-driven insights. Medical Professionals may also explore the potential of AI in predictive analytics for early detection of nutritional deficiencies and disease risk factors, leading to proactive interventions for improved longevity.

NAME: Public Health Experts
BELIEVE: Public Health Experts recognize the potential of AI to address population-level challenges in promoting healthy eating habits and preventing chronic diseases. They believe that AI-powered analytics inform targeted interventions and policies to improve nutritional outcomes across diverse communities. Public Health Experts value the scalability and efficiency of AI in processing large datasets to identify trends and disparities in nutrition-related health outcomes.

COUNTERING CRITICS: Public Health Experts defend their use of AI by emphasizing the focus on population health and equity in their approach to nutrition-driven longevity. They argue that AI helps overcome logistical barriers and resource constraints in public health initiatives, leading to more effective and sustainable interventions. Public Health Experts stress the importance of community engagement and interdisciplinary collaboration to ensure that AI strategies are culturally sensitive and contextually relevant.

EVOLVING TO 2030: In the year 2030, Public Health Experts may use AI technologies to develop predictive models for evaluating the impact of nutrition interventions on population health outcomes. They could harness machine learning algorithms to customize public health campaigns and initiatives based on demographic and socioeconomic factors. Public Health Experts may also advocate for the ethical and transparent use of AI in public health decision-making to uphold principles of social justice and health equity.

NAME: Nutrition Scientists
BELIEVE: Nutrition Scientists view AI as a powerful tool for advancing research in precision nutrition and personalized dietary recommendations. They believe that AI analyzes complex interactions between nutrients, genetic factors, and health outcomes to inform evidence-based guidelines for optimal longevity. Nutritional Scientists recognize the potential of AI to streamline data analysis and hypothesis testing in nutrition research, accelerating scientific discoveries and breakthroughs.

COUNTERING CRITICS: Nutrition Scientists defend their integration of AI by highlighting the rigorous validation and peer review processes inherent in their research methodologies. They emphasize the importance of transparency and reproducibility in AI-driven studies to ensure scientific integrity and credibility. Nutrition Scientists underscore the need for interdisciplinary collaboration and data sharing to maximize the impact of AI in advancing nutrition science.

EVOLVING TO 2030: By 2030, Nutrition Scientists may adopt cutting-edge AI technologies, such as deep learning and natural language processing, to extract valuable insights from vast amounts of scientific literature and clinical data. They could develop AI-powered predictive models for assessing individual dietary responses and monitoring long-term health outcomes. Nutrition Scientists may also explore the integration of AI with emerging technologies, such as blockchain and Internet of Things (IoT), to create secure and decentralized platforms for nutrition research and collaboration.

Table 3.
Two groups of four mind-sets each (general professional, nutrition profession) as simulated by AI.

5. Focus 4: Analysis of viewpoints regarding incorporating AI in the nutrition-longevity link

The incorporation of AI nutrition and longevity has elicited diverse reactions from various groups. Experts regard AI as a potent instrument for examining and enhancing dietary habits aimed at fostering longevity and improving overall health. Yet, some raise alarms regarding the ethical ramifications of AI influencing dietary advice. Skeptics express concern that an overreliance on AI algorithms could simplify the intricate nature of nutritional needs and overlook personal variations. Conversely, supporters contend that AI can precisely customize dietary plans by considering genetic factors, lifestyle habits, and disease risks.

Different health organizations, such as the World Health Organization and the American Heart Association, have expressed varying views on the role of AI in the connection between nutrition and longevity. Consumer advocacy groups have expressed concerns regarding the transparency and accountability of AI-driven nutrition products and services. Public sentiment regarding AI in nutrition and longevity is polarized; some individuals welcome its promising advantages, while others advocate for increased regulation and oversight. The perspectives of various groups offer important insights into the changing dynamics of AI, nutrition, and longevity.

Table 4 shows how the AI embedded in the Mind Genomics platform, BimiLeap.com (Idea Coach feature), provides critical thinking regarding viewpoints about AI in nutritional science. The Mind Genomics platform is set up to provide various "analyses" of data simulation. One of these analyses looks at "viewpoints," including those who are positive about AI in nutrition, those who oppose AI in nutrition, and "out-of-the-box thinking" under the rubric of "alternative viewpoints."

---

1 INTERESTED AUDIENCES

1. *Health and wellness enthusiasts:* Individuals who are interested in maintaining a healthy lifestyle and maximizing their longevity would be keen to learn about how food preferences influence their lifespan, as well as specific dietary patterns and foods that support longevity. They may also be interested in personalized recommendations based on genetic factors to optimize their diet for longevity.
2. *Medical professionals*: Healthcare providers, nutritionists, and dietitians benefit from understanding the insights provided by AI on food preferences and longevity outcomes. This knowledge helps them tailor dietary recommendations for their patients to support overall health and wellness.
3. *Researchers and scientists*: Professionals in the field of nutrition, longevity research, and artificial intelligence find value in the topic questions as they explore the intersection of food preferences, genetics, and health outcomes. AI analysis provides new insights and drives additional research in this area.
4. *Public health officials*: Policymakers and public health professionals may be interested in understanding the impact of socioeconomic factors on food preferences and longevity outcomes. This information informs strategies to address health disparities and promote healthier eating habits among different populations.
5. *Individuals interested in preventive health*: Those who prioritize preventive health measures to avoid chronic diseases and enhance their quality of life would find the insights from AI analysis on longevity and food preferences, particularly valuable. This information helps them make informed choices to optimize their diet for longevity and overall wellness.

2 OPPOSING AUDIENCES

1. *Traditionalists:* Some individuals who adhere to traditional dietary beliefs or cultural practices may be resistant to incorporating AI recommendations into their lifestyle. They may view AI analysis as undermining their cultural heritage or personal beliefs about food and longevity.
2. *Skeptics of technology*: People who are wary of artificial intelligence and its potential impact on human health and well-being may be hesitant to trust AI recommendations on food preferences and longevity. They may have concerns about privacy, accuracy, or ethical implications of using AI in this context.

---

3. *Industry stakeholders*: Companies in the food and beverage industry that produce and market products that may not align with AI recommendations for longevity may oppose the topic. They may fear that AI analysis could lead to consumer backlash against certain products or result in changes to industry regulations.
4. *Individuals with conflicting interests*: People who have financial interests in promoting certain dietary products or practices that are not supported by AI analysis may oppose the topic. They may perceive AI recommendations as a threat to their business or personal agenda.
5. *Those resistant to change*: Some individuals who are resistant to change or prefer to stick to familiar habits and routines may resist adopting AI recommendations for optimizing their diet for longevity. They may be comfortable with their current dietary choices and reluctant to make changes based on AI insights.

3 ALTERNATIVE (OUT OF THE BOX) VIEWPOINTS

1. Some may argue that genetics play a greater role in longevity than dietary preferences, and that individuals are predisposed to certain health outcomes regardless of their food choices.
2. There may be skepticism towards AI's ability to provide accurate recommendations for optimal longevity, with concerns about the reliability of data and the potential for bias in analysis.
3. Critics may believe that superfoods are overhyped and that a well-rounded diet with moderation is more important for overall health and longevity than focusing on specific "miracle" foods.
4. Some individuals may prioritize taste and enjoyment in their food preferences over longevity outcomes, believing that life is meant to be lived to the fullest rather than strictly controlled through diet.
5. Cultural and societal factors may influence food preferences and longevity outcomes in ways that AI analysis may not fully capture, leading to potential gaps in understanding the complex relationship between diet and lifespan.
6. There may be disagreement on the role of gut health in promoting longevity, with some questioning the importance of the microbiome in overall health and wellness.
7. Skeptics may argue that AI's personalized dietary recommendations based on genetics are overly simplistic and fail to consider the broader environmental and lifestyle factors that contribute to longevity.
8. Critics may point out that socioeconomic disparities in access to healthy foods and resources are deeply entrenched and require systemic change beyond individual dietary choices to address effectively.
9. Some may question the accuracy and validity of AI predictions on future trends in food preferences and longevity outcomes, arguing that unforeseen variables could affect the reliability of such forecasts.
10. Alternative viewpoints may emphasize the importance of balance, variety, and enjoyment in diet rather than strict adherence to specific recommendations for longevity, highlighting the individual nature of dietary preferences and choices.

Table 4.
The three types of audiences involved in AI in nutrition: Interested audiences, opposing audiences, and alternative viewpoints.

6. Focus 5: Critical thinking to identify themes and perspectives

Through the exploration of various themes and viewpoints, AI unveils distinctive insights into intricate matters. AI sifts through data, extracting insights and making informed decisions grounded in evidence and logic (see **Table 5**). This method enables AI to explore various perspectives and possible solutions to an issue. AI uncovers patterns and trends often missed by humans, enhancing the efficiency of problem-solving. AI, through critical thinking, questions established beliefs and uncovers fresh opportunities. AI adjusts its reasoning in response to new information

Critical thinking—analysis of themes from different perspective

1. Influence of Food Preferences on Longevity
   - The influence of food preferences on longevity outcomes as analyzed by AI
   - The impact of superfoods on lifespan based on AI research findings
   - Predicting future trends in food preferences and their implications for longevity outcomes using AI
     - o *Plus*: AI provides valuable data and insights to help individuals make more informed choices about their diet and potentially improve their longevity.
     - o *Minus*: Potential limitations in the accuracy and reliability of AI predictions regarding the impact of food preferences on longevity outcomes.
     - o *Interesting*: The use of AI technology to analyze large amounts of data and identify patterns that may not be immediately apparent to humans.
2. Recommended Dietary Patterns for Longevity
   - Specific dietary patterns recommended by AI for promoting longevity
   - AI recommendations for maintaining a healthy weight to support longevity
   - Improving brain health and cognitive function through dietary choices according to AI analysis
     - o *Plus*: AI analyzes complex datasets to determine the most effective dietary patterns for promoting longevity.
     - o *Minus*: Limitations in the ability of AI to account for individual variability in response to different dietary patterns.
     - o *Interesting*: The potential for AI to continuously adapt and refine dietary recommendations based on real-time data and feedback.
3. Personalized Nutrition for Longevity
   - Providing personalized dietary recommendations based on an individual's genetic profile for optimizing longevity
     - o *Plus*: Personalized dietary recommendations based on genetic analysis potentially lead to more tailored and effective strategies for promoting longevity.
     - o *Minus*: Concerns about the privacy and ethical implications of using genetic information to inform dietary recommendations.
     - o *Interesting*: The intersection of AI technology and genetics in optimizing nutrition for longevity.
4. Gut Health and Longevity
   - The importance of gut health in promoting longevity as recognized by AI
     - o *Plus*: AI helps identify the role of gut health in promoting longevity and suggests dietary strategies to support a healthy gut microbiome.
     - o *Minus*: Challenges in accurately assessing and interpreting the impact of gut health on longevity outcomes using AI.
     - o *Interesting*: The potential for AI to uncover new connections between gut health and longevity through advanced data analysis.
5. Socioeconomic Factors and Longevity
   - Insights from AI research on the impact of socioeconomic factors on food preferences and longevity outcomes
     - o *Plus*: AI research sheds light on the complex relationship between socioeconomic factors, food preferences, and longevity outcomes.
     - o *Minus*: Risks of oversimplifying the influence of socioeconomic factors on longevity outcomes without considering individual experiences and circumstances.
     - o *Interesting*: The potential for AI to uncover hidden disparities and inequalities in access to healthy food and resources that impact longevity.

6. Strategies for Optimizing Diet for Longevity

- Strategies individuals adopt based on AI insights to optimize their diet for longevity and overall health
  - o *Plus*: AI insights empower individuals to make more informed choices about their diet and lifestyle to support longevity.
  - o *Minus*: Potential challenges in implementing and sustaining dietary changes based on AI recommendations.
  - o *Interesting*: The innovative approaches and technologies that are used to support individuals in optimizing their diet for longevity.

Table 5.
Six "themes" and then perspectives about those themes, suggested by AI regarding nutrition and longevity.

and feedback, enhancing its capacity to analyze problems. The critical thinking skills of AI allow it to maneuver through ambiguity and uncertainty, establishing it as an invaluable asset for decision-making across diverse domains.

7. Focus 6: AI-suggested process innovations for nutrition to increase longevity

AI's capacity to sift through extensive data and make instantaneous decisions allows companies to enhance efficiency, cut expenses, and provide healthier food choices. Innovations in processes that blend AI with nutrition may transform food production, distribution, and consumption, enhancing manufacturing processes, elevating food quality and safety, and crafting tailored nutrition solutions. These innovations increase efficiency and productivity while prioritizing the health and well-being of consumers. **Table 6** shows five innovations in food and nutrition to enhance longevity as first suggested by AI and further analyzed by AI.

1. *Personalized meal delivery services that use AI algorithms to create customized meal plans based on an individual's dietary preferences, health goals, and genetic profile for promoting longevity.*
   SUGGESTION: By tailoring meal plans to each person's unique needs, this service enhances overall health and well-being. The incorporation of genetic profiles helps to further individualize the meal plans, ensuring that individuals receive the nutrients their bodies require. Ultimately, this could lead to improved longevity and disease prevention, as individuals are provided with precisely what their bodies need to thrive.
   STRATEGY TO GET THE INNOVATION ACCEPTED: Offer a free trial period or discounted introductory offer. This would allow individuals to experience the convenience and benefits of having customized meal plans tailored to their specific needs without fully committing them upfront. Additionally, providing educational resources and support from nutritionists or dietitians to help users understand the science behind the personalized meal plans and how it benefits their health and longevity could also incentivize people to invest in the service. Giving users the option to personalize and adjust their meal plans based on their feedback and results further enhances the value proposition and makes it more appealing for potential investors.
2. *Nutritional supplements designed specifically to target key biomarkers associated with aging and longevity, based on AI analysis of optimal nutrient intake for longevity.*
   SUGGESTION: By using AI to analyze optimal nutrient intake for longevity, these supplements could potentially enhance cellular function, reduce inflammation, and improve overall health markers associated with aging. This targeted approach may also help individuals prevent age-related diseases and maintain vitality as they grow older. Ultimately, this innovation could revolutionize the field of anti-aging and lead to a more personalized and effective approach to promoting longevity.

STRATEGY TO GET THE INNOVATION ACCEPTED: Offer personalized recommendations based on individual health assessments. By incorporating AI analysis to determine each person's unique nutrient needs, individuals may be more willing to invest in supplements that are tailored to their specific biomarkers and health goals. Additionally, providing evidence-based research on the effectiveness of these supplements in extending lifespan and improving overall health may also incentivize individuals to consider investing in this idea. By showing individuals the personalized benefits and potential outcomes of these supplements, they may be more inclined to invest in their health and longevity.
3. *AI-powered mobile apps which track an individual's food intake, analyze dietary patterns, and provide real-time feedback and recommendations for improving longevity through better nutrition.* *SUGGESTION*: By using AI technology, people receive personalized insights into their food intake and make more informed decisions about their dietary habits. With real-time feedback and recommendations, users easily identify areas for improvement and tailor their eating habits to support longevity and overall health. This innovative approach could empower individuals to take control of their well-being and make sustainable changes to optimize their nutrition for a longer, healthier life. *STRATEGY TO GET THE INNOVATION ACCEPTED*: Offer a free trial period or a discounted subscription rate for a limited time. This would allow users to try out the app and experience the benefits firsthand before committing to a full-price subscription. Additionally, offering personalized discounts or rewards for achieving certain health or nutrition goals through the app could provide further incentives for users to invest in the technology. By making the app more accessible and rewarding for users, they are more likely to see the value in investing in their long-term health and nutrition.
4. *Virtual reality experiences that simulate the benefits of a healthy diet for longevity, guiding users through immersive scenarios that illustrate the impact* of food choices on aging and lifespan. *SUGGESTION*: By immersing users in virtual reality scenarios that showcase the effects of different foods on aging and lifespan, they gain a better understanding of the importance of nutrition for longevity. This hands-on approach may make it easier for individuals to make healthier food choices in their daily lives, leading to improved overall health and potentially extending their lifespan. Ultimately, this innovative use of technology could help combat the increasing rates of chronic diseases associated with poor dietary habits. *STRATEGY TO GET THE INNOVATION ACCEPTED*: Offer a free trial or a discounted rate for the virtual reality experience for a limited time, allowing users to try out the program and see the potential benefits before committing to a full purchase. Additionally, providing evidence-based research and testimonials from experts in nutrition and longevity could help convince skeptics of the effectiveness of the program. A money-back guarantee could also give users peace of mind that they are making a risk-free investment in their health and longevity. By combining these strategies, more people may be willing to invest in the virtual reality experience and take control of their dietary choices for a healthier and longer life.
5. *Policy initiatives that utilize AI to analyze population-level data on food preferences, nutritional intake, and longevity outcomes to inform public health recommendations and interventions aimed at promoting healthier dietary habits for longevity.* *SUGGESTION*: Implementing policy initiatives that use AI to analyze population-level data on food preferences, nutritional intake, and longevity outcomes have implications for public health. By using AI, policymakers gain valuable insights into the factors that contribute to healthier dietary habits and longevity, allowing for more targeted and effective interventions. This approach identifies trends and patterns in dietary choices, allowing for the development of personalized recommendations tailored to specific demographics. Ultimately, this reduces chronic diseases and an improvement in overall population health and longevity. *STRATEGY TO GET THE INNOVATION ACCEPTED*: Offer incentives or rewards for participating in data collection and analysis. This could include offering discounts on healthy food options, access to personalized nutrition plans or consultations, or even monetary rewards for contributing to the research. Additionally, emphasizing the potential benefits of adopting healthier dietary habits for longevity, such as improved quality of life, reduced risk of chronic diseases, and increased lifespan, could motivate individuals to participate in and support these initiatives. Ultimately, by demonstrating the tangible value and impact of using AI for public health interventions, people may be more willing to invest in this idea.

Table 6.
Five process innovations suggested by AI for nutrition to increase longevity.

8. Focus 7: Using AI to pose relevant questions and generate answers

The final focus or topic is the use of AI to teach in the Socratic fashion by posing questions and providing answers. AI-generated questions and answers support education and research. AI's proficiency in natural language processing and contextual understanding enables it to deliver answers that are both personalized and relevant to inquiries. Concerns have emerged regarding the accuracy and bias present in AI-generated responses. However, as AI evolves, the significance and complexity of AI-generated questions and answers are likely to become more "correct" and useful, as the factors leading to the distortion of information are discovered and dealt with appropriately. **Table** 7 shows five questions and answers generated by AI, to give a sense of the type of teaching which can emerge from the creation of a dialog through questions and answers.

QUESTION 1: How does AI help individuals make more informed choices about their dietary habits to increase their lifespan?
AI in nutrition empowers individuals to make choices that support longevity and overall wellness. AI helps individuals make more informed choices about their dietary habits by analyzing personal health data, nutritional needs, and preferences to provide personalized recommendations. By incorporating machine learning algorithms, AI tracks and analyzes dietary patterns, metabolism, and genetic information to offer tailored guidance on what foods to eat or avoid. AI also monitors individuals' progress, adjusts recommendations as needed, and provide timely reminders or alerts to promote adherence to healthy eating habits. Additionally, AI-powered apps and devices offer real-time feedback on food choices, portion sizes, and nutritional content to help users make better decisions about their diet.

QUESTION 2: What ethical considerations should be considered when using AI to study nutrition and longevity?
When using AI to study nutrition and longevity, several ethical considerations must be addressed to ensure that data privacy, consent, bias, and accountability are upheld. It is essential to protect individuals' personal information and ensure that data collected for research purposes is anonymized and securely stored to prevent unauthorized access or misuse. Additionally, researchers must obtain informed consent from participants and clearly communicate the goals, risks, and potential benefits of the study involving AI technology. Moreover, efforts should be made to mitigate bias in AI algorithms by monitoring bias, ensuring diverse training data sets, and providing transparency in the decision-making process. Lastly, accountability mechanisms should be put in place to address any unintended consequences or ethical breaches that may arise from using AI in nutrition and longevity studies.

QUESTION 3: How does AI help healthcare professionals better understand the impact of diets on longevity and overall health?
AI helps healthcare professionals better understand the impact of diets on longevity and overall health by processing vast amounts of data, identifying patterns, and generating insights that may not be readily apparent through traditional methods. By analyzing electronic health records, genetic information, dietary intake, and clinical outcomes, AI uncovers correlations between diets and health outcomes, identifies risk factors for certain diseases, and predicts individualized responses to different dietary interventions. Moreover, AI facilitates large-scale observational studies, clinical trials, and meta-analyses to advance our understanding of the complex relationships between diet, lifestyle factors, and longevity. By using AI tools and technologies, healthcare professionals make evidence-based recommendations, develop personalized treatment plans, and monitor patients' progress to optimize their overall health and well-being.

QUESTION 4: How does AI identify potential dietary interventions that may help individuals live longer and healthier lives?
AI analyzes a wide range of factors, such as genetic predispositions, metabolic profiles, environmental influences, and lifestyle habits. Through data mining techniques, AI discovers novel correlations between specific nutrients, foods, or dietary patterns and various health outcomes, such as reduced risk of chronic diseases, improved metabolic health, and enhanced longevity. By integrating multiple sources of information, including biological markers, dietary assessments, and clinical data, AI generates

personalized recommendations for dietary changes, supplementation, or behavioral modifications that align with individuals' unique needs and goals. Additionally, AI-powered algorithms continuously learn and adapt based on new data, emerging research, and individual responses to interventions, allowing for more targeted, effective, and sustainable dietary strategies to support long-term health and well-being.

QUESTION 5: What advancements in AI technology are needed to further enhance our understanding of the relationship between longevity and food preferences, nutrition, and attitudes towards food?
To further enhance our understanding of the relationship between longevity and food preferences, nutrition, and attitudes towards food, advancements in AI technology are needed in several key areas. First, there is a need for more sophisticated algorithms that analyze complex, multifaceted data sets, including genomic, microbiome, behavioral, and environmental data, to uncover deeper insights into the factors influencing dietary choices, metabolic processes, and health outcomes. Second, AI tools that integrate data from multiple sources, such as wearable devices, food tracking apps, and medical records, in real-time are essential for capturing dynamic changes in individuals' dietary patterns and health status over time. Third, the development of explainable AI models that transparently interpret and communicate the rationale behind recommendations related to food choices, nutrition, and longevity is crucial for building trust, fostering engagement, and supporting informed decision-making by users and healthcare professionals. Lastly, ongoing advancements in AI research, including reinforcement learning, natural language processing, and causal inference, help address the complexity and uncertainty inherent in studying the intricate interactions between nutrition, longevity, and human behavior, paving the way for more personalized, effective, and sustainable strategies for promoting health and well-being through diet.

Table 7.
Five AI-generated questions and answers dealing with nutrition and longevity.

9. Discussion and conclusions

Artificial intelligence (AI) plays an increasingly important role in the field of nutrition today by using algorithms to analyze data related to genetic information, dietary habits, and lifestyle factors. This allows experts to identify patterns and correlations that may impact overall health and lifespan. By providing personalized nutrition recommendations based on individual needs and goals, AI helps optimize nutrient intake and minimize deficiencies. AI also assists in predicting and preventing chronic diseases by analyzing various risk factors and developing targeted interventions. This technology can aid in meal planning, tracking, and monitoring to ensure individuals meet their nutritional needs and health goals. Furthermore, AI contributes to the development of innovative nutritional supplements and functional foods that target specific health concerns and promote longevity. Research in precision nutrition is also advancing thanks to AI, providing real-time feedback and monitoring of an individual's nutritional status and health markers. Overall, the integration of AI in nutrition holds great promise for advancing the understanding of how nutrition can drive longevity and help individuals live longer, healthier lives.

Acknowledgements

The paper was written in a cooperative fashion with ChatGPT 3.5 embedded in the Mind Genomics platform, BimiLeap.com (Idea Coach feature).

The authors wish to thank Vanessa Marie B. Arcenas and Angela A. for their efforts in preparing this and other manuscripts for publication.

Author details

Howard R. Moskowitz[1,2]* and Sharon Wingert[1]

1 Tactical Data Group, Stafford, VA, USA

2 Mind Genomics Associates, Inc., White Plains, NY, USA

*Address all correspondence to: mjihrm@gmail.com

References

[1] Côté M, Lamarche B. Artificial intelligence in nutrition research: Perspectives on current and future applications. Applied Physiology, Nutrition, and Metabolism. 2022;**47**(1): 1-8. DOI: 10.1139/apnm-2021-0448

[2] Limketkai BN, Mauldin K, Manitius N, Jalilian L, Salonen BR. The age of artificial intelligence: Use of digital technology in clinical nutrition. Current Surgery Reports. 2021;**9**(7):20. DOI: 10.1007/s40137-021-00297-3

[3] Miyazawa T, Hiratsuka Y, Toda M, Hatakeyama N, Ozawa H, Abe C, et al. Artificial intelligence in food science and nutrition: A narrative review. Nutrition Reviews. 2022;**80**(12):2288-2300. DOI: 10.1093/nutrit/nuac033

[4] Sosa-Holwerda A, Park OH, Albracht-Schulte K, Niraula S, Thompson L, Oldewage-Theron W. The role of artificial intelligence in nutrition research: A scoping review. Nutrients. 2024;**16**(13):2066. DOI: 10.3390/nu16132066

[5] Honka A, Kaipainen K, Hietala H, Saranummi N. Rethinking health: ICT-enabled services to empower people to manage their health. IEEE Reviews in Biomedical Engineering. 2011;**4**:119-139. DOI: 10.1109/RBME.2011.2174217

[6] Fadhil A, Gabrielli S. Addressing challenges in promoting healthy lifestyles: The al-chatbot approach. In: Proceedings of the 11th EAI International Conference on Pervasive Computing Technologies for Healthcare. 2017. pp. 261-265. DOI: 10.1145/3154862.3154914

[7] Woods T. Live longer with AI: How Artificial Intelligence Is Helping us Extend our Healthspan and Live Better Too. Birmingham: Packt Publishing Ltd; 2020

[8] Young S. The Science and Technology of Growing Young, Updated Edition: An Insider's Guide to the Breakthroughs That Will Dramatically Extend our Lifespan ... and What you Can Do Right Now. Dallas: BenBella Books; 2024

[9] Finch CE. The Biology of Human Longevity: Inflammation, Nutrition, and Aging in the Evolution of Lifespans. 1st ed. San Diego: Academic Press; 2010

[10] Iwendi C, Khan S, Anajemba JH, Bashir AK, Noor F. Realizing an efficient IoMT-assisted patient diet recommendation system through machine learning model. IEEE Access. 2020;**8**:28462-28474. DOI: 10.1109/ACCESS.2020.2968537

[11] Ohlhorst SD, Russell R, Bier D, Klurfeld DM, Li Z, Mein JR, et al. Nutrition research to affect food and a healthy lifespan. Advances in Nutrition. 2013;**4**(5):579-584. DOI: 10.3945/an.113.004176

[12] Bush CL, Blumberg JB, El-Sohemy A, Minich DM, Ordovás JM, Reed DG, et al. Toward the definition of personalized nutrition: A proposal by the American nutrition association. Journal of the American College of Nutrition. 2020;**39**(1):5-15. DOI: 10.1080/07315724.2019.1685332

[13] Topol E. Deep Medicine: How Artificial Intelligence Can Make Healthcare Human Again. New York: Basic Books; 2019

[14] Dias SB, Oikonomidis Y, Diniz JA, Baptista F, Carnide F, Bensenousi A, et al. Users' perspective on the AI-based

smartphone PROTEIN app for personalized nutrition and healthy living: A modified technology acceptance model (mTAM) approach. Frontiers in Nutrition. 2022;**9**:898031. DOI: 10.3389/fnut.2022.898031

[15] Huang CY, Yang MC. Empirical investigation of factors influencing consumer intention to use an artificial intelligence-powered mobile application for weight loss and health management. Telemedicine and E-Health. 2020; **26**(10):1240-1251. DOI: 10.1089/tmj.2019.0182

[16] Vasiloglou MF, Christodoulidis S, Reber E, Stathopoulou T, Lu Y, Stanga Z, et al. What healthcare professionals think of "nutrition and diet" apps: An international survey. Nutrients. 2020; **12**(8):2214. DOI: doi.org/10.3390/nu12082214

[17] Young AT, Amara D, Bhattacharya A, Wei ML. Patient and general public attitudes towards clinical artificial intelligence: A mixed methods systematic review. The Lancet Digital Health. 2021;**3**(9):e599-e611

[18] Dweck CS, Yeager DS. Mindsets: A view from two eras. Perspectives on Psychological Science. 2019;**14**(3): 481-496. DOI: 10.1177/1745691618804166

[19] Hamilton R, Vohs KD, Sellier AL, Meyvis T. Being of two minds: Switching mindsets exhausts self-regulatory resources. Organizational Behavior and Human Decision Processes. 2011;**115**(1): 13-24. DOI: 10.1016/j.obhdp.2010.11.005

[20] Moskowitz H. 'Diabesity'–using mind genomics thinking coupled with AI to synthesize mind-sets and provide direction for changing behavior. American Journal of Medical and Clinical Research and Reviews. 2024;**3**(3):1-3. DOI: 10.58372/2835-6276.1148

[21] Moskowitz HR, Rappaport SD, Saharan S, Wingert S, Anderson T, Mulvey T, et al. Mind-sets for prescription weight loss products that are advertised directly to consumers: Using mind genomics thinking with AI for synthesis and exploration. Acta Scientific Pharmaceutical Sciences (ISSN: 2581–5423). 2024;**8**(6):80-87. DOI: 10.31080/ASPS.2024.08.1072

[22] Orvidas K, Burnette JL, Schleider JL, Skelton JA, Moses M, Dunsmore JC. Healthy body, healthy mind: A mindset intervention for obese youth. The Journal of Genetic Psychology. 2020; **181**(6):443-457. DOI: 10.1080/00221325.2020.1796573

Chapter 10

Quality of Life in People Living with Dementia: Personalized Early Diagnosis, Individual Empowerment, and Community Inclusion

Francesca Morganti

Abstract

The quality of life for individuals living with dementia appears to be a significant challenge. To date, the determinants that play a key role in maximizing their daily life have not been highlighted, remaining a widely neglected area of scientific study and intervention. This contribution focuses on elements that are most likely to lead people who are on the verge of aging toward quality aging despite dementia, considering that individuals are capable of shaping, influencing, or regulating their own trajectory throughout their lifespan. A fundamental premise of this proposal is the notion that an individual's capacity to regulate their own growth and development over the course of their life determines their overall well-being, and that trajectories of dementia can be classified as "successful" or "unsuccessful" based on this regulatory process. The proposal outlines specific actions aimed at fostering well-being throughout the dementia process, including the early diagnosis of dementia, the empowerment of individuals during their lifespan, and the creation of a dementia-friendly community that ensures full participation in everyday activities. These actions are intended to enhance and maximize dementia pathways. The implementation of these strategies necessitates a cultural transformation concerning the perception of dementia. Illustrative examples of this cultural shift will be drawn from the recent research conducted in the Bergamo region.

Keywords: aging with dementia, quality of life, empowerment, early diagnosis, dementia-friendly, ageism

1. Introduction

While it is not asserted that dementia is an inherent aspect of the aging process, it is noteworthy that the prevalence of dementia is notably high among the elderly population. In numerous instances, dementia has been observed to contribute to a decline in the quality of life and autonomy of individuals affected by the condition. It is, therefore, imperative to recognize that while the third age is characterized as the period of life in which individuals are predisposed to developing pathologies that lead to states of frailty and dependency, aging can still be seen as a period in the life cycle, in which the potential of the individual can be used to ensure that this stage is characterized by "quality" in itself. This assertion is substantiated by the observation that the older population experiencing frailty is disproportionately susceptible to cognitive diseases, such as dementia, compared to their non-frail counterparts [1]. Therefore, it is imperative to closely examine frailty and its potential impact on the deterioration of cognitive function, especially in the context of its role in increasing the risk of developing dementia [2].

Recently, Wallace et al. identified a role for frailty in the association between Alzheimer's disease and related dementias [3]. Although in any case it is still unclear whether the association between frailty and Alzheimer's disease pathophysiology is due to direct mechanisms (e.g., amyloid pathology causes frailty) or indirect mechanisms (e.g., amyloid pathology and frailty are linked in that they are both age-related), this study asks us to consider how frailty may represent a potentially modifiable focus for early cognitive impairment. This underscores its capacity for early and "tailored" clinical intervention. The assessment of frailty in clinical practice has become a useful tool for healthcare professionals, such as psychologists, educators, and geriatricians. By utilizing this assessment, professionals can personalize interventions to support individuals in maintaining a healthy state of frailty or to provide therapeutic interventions in cases of pathological decline. Indeed, the identification of frailty should prompt professionals to undertake a more precise investigation of the determinants that contribute to an individual's increased vulnerability and that may lead to the development of dementia, given its prevalence in the elderly population. This approach enables the adoption of a person-centered treatment strategy aimed at mitigating potential adverse outcomes and disrupting the prevailing paradigm of aging as synonymous with the accrual of diseases.

As a result, in contemporary discourse, the construct of frailty is increasingly used as a measure of an individual's risk profile, thus it plays a significant role in determining an individual's biological aging profile. This is predicated on the premise that chronological age may not always correspond to biological progression. Consequently, it provides a framework for understanding aging as having infinite trajectories, potentially following different profiles of frailty or eventual pathology.

The aforementioned perspective redefines the aged population as extremely heterogeneous. Consequently, a comprehensive evaluation of specific aging individuals, with the objective of early detection of potential pathological profiles, can only be achieved by integrating the construct of frailty with another crucial concept: the biological and cognitive reserve accumulated throughout the lifespan [4]. In particular, the potential countermeasures available to date to mitigate dementia include the personalization of empowerment strategies to support the aging individual in their future life trajectory. This approach acknowledges the wealth of experiences, skills, and relationships accumulated throughout one's life and seeks to foster a fulfilling relationship with the context in which the individual lives, including the trajectory of dementia [5]. This approach is essential to ensure a meaningful experience for the person and to maximize their quality of life, and to ensure a fruitful relationship with the context in which the person operates in any trajectory, including that of dementia pathology.

2. Reconsidering the neural and cognitive reserve in frailty and dementia

Considering lifespan trajectories, among the theories that highlight neural and cognitive reserve as critical determinants of successful aging, the neural maintenance theory posits that older individuals with a well-preserved nervous system are also those who demonstrate optimized cognitive functioning as they age [6]. While neural maintenance may appear to be an advantageous mechanism, it is important to acknowledge that the majority of the elderly population inevitably experiences age-related brain atrophy [7]. Nevertheless, it is well established that some individuals can successfully perform cognitive tasks by engaging in what are referred to as compensatory processes [8].

Emphasizing the complexity of aging, it is crucial to recognize that individuals may not only exhibit varying degrees of brain atrophy but also differ in their ability to deploy compensatory strategies of varying effectiveness. These strategies are shaped by cognitive reserve, which in turn is influenced by an individual's unique life history and experiences.

To theoretically delineate the interplay between frailty, neural reserve, and cognitive reserve, we can argue that even when two older adults exhibit identical neural changes, one may demonstrate lower levels of frailty in daily life due to a greater cognitive reserve and more effective compensatory mechanisms. Conversely, from a speculative standpoint, marked age-related brain atrophy, when coupled with a weak compensatory capacity, may be indicative of a trajectory toward pathological cognitive decline [9]. Examples of such conditions include mild cognitive impairment (MCI) or mild neurocognitive disorder [10], as well as more severe neurodegenerative conditions, now classified as major neurocognitive disorders [11].

As in all developmental and learning trajectories, aging involves a synergistic interplay between biological factors (e.g., genetic predisposition) and environmental influences (e.g., lifestyle). Both factors are presumed to shape cognitive performance in aging by influencing the extent of age-related neural changes (such as the maintenance or atrophy of the nervous system) and the ability to employ compensatory strategies. For instance, being a carrier of a genetic variation, such as the APOE ε4 allele, has been linked to an increased risk of hippocampal atrophy in aging [12]. At the same time, a low level of education has been associated with reduced cognitive reserve and diminished compensatory capacity [13, 14].

There is considerable heterogeneity in the structure and function of the nervous system among older adults, which contributes to distinct trajectories of cognitive decline, frailty, and successful aging. Neuroimaging studies have highlighted significant interindividual differences in structural aging, evident in white matter hyperintensities, interhemispheric connectivity, and cortical and subcortical volume changes. Such findings have led to the conceptualization of "Δ brain age"—the discrepancy between an individual's chronological age and their brain age [15]. A positive Δ suggests accelerated brain aging, whereas a negative Δ indicates a well-preserved nervous system [16].

Given this complexity, frailty is now understood not only as a biological construct but also as the outcome of interactions between an individual's physical and cognitive abilities and their environmental context [17]. Thus, interventions aimed at optimizing functional ability in aging, including in pathological conditions, should focus on enhancing reserves and mitigating frailty. This necessitates comprehensive assessments that extend beyond the individual to their living environment, where challenges to frailty or dementia-related conditions may arise.

A lifespan perspective underscores the need for a dynamic and adaptive approach to aging, accommodating diverse trajectories ranging from healthy aging to frailty and dementia. Tracking an individual's life course allows for targeted interventions and the implementation of educational programs that foster inclusion within their community. Such efforts can support developmental trajectories, either before or during the onset of dementia-related symptoms.

As individuals age, their abilities fluctuate, making their interaction with the environment increasingly complex. Therefore, person-centered interventions should move beyond a compensatory and assistive framework toward empowering older adults, particularly those with dementia. Rather than solely mitigating cognitive decline, the goal should be to support their independence and enable them to continue engaging in personal interests and social roles. This approach not only fosters active participation in society but also contributes to reversing frailty trajectories over the lifespan. By accumulating cognitive and neural reserves, individuals may not necessarily prevent dementia onset but can better cope with its progression, maintaining an optimal quality of life.

From a clinical perspective, diagnosis and treatment of dementia should prioritize proactive strategies that encourage individuals to take early responsibility for their psychophysical well-being across the lifespan. Early identification of cognitive decline and dementia risk enables the development of personalized care plans tailored to an individual's values and priorities [18]. The objective is not merely to slow excessive cognitive decline but, more importantly, to ensure the highest possible quality of life for aging individuals.

3. Counteracting ageism and on the road toward an early diagnosis: The entitlement to quality of life in dementia

The conceptualization of dementia outlined above often encounters significant barriers to its practical implementation. One of the foremost challenges lies in confronting culturally ingrained perceptions of aging, commonly referred to as ageism [19]. This widespread stereotype predominantly portrays older individuals as retreating from productive life, experiencing progressive declines in autonomy, and requiring increasing levels of support. Such a perspective not only marginalizes older adults—especially those who are frail or living with pathological aging—but also profoundly impacts their capacity for self-determination and empowerment, thereby diminishing their overall quality of life.

A closer examination of older individuals reveals how meanings attributed to aging are deeply shaped by cultural contexts, influencing how older people perceive themselves. Empirical research consistently demonstrates that individuals, often unconsciously, internalize these negative stereotypes. As a result, older adults tend to adopt more sedentary lifestyles, underestimate their cognitive abilities, and become entangled in a cycle of physical and mental decline. These factors collectively contribute to a reduced lifespan [20]. The public health consequences of ageism are profound, leading to an increased prevalence of cardiovascular diseases, chronic respiratory conditions, and diabetes mellitus, with significant economic burdens on healthcare systems [21].

The impact of ageism becomes even more pronounced in the context of dementia. Ageism serves as a powerful and detrimental force, as individuals may simultaneously be both perpetrators and victims of ageist behaviors. On the one hand, older adults with dementia often face social exclusion, distrust, or patronizing treatment (e.g., being perceived as incompetent, forgetful, or burdensome). On the other hand, they may internalize these attitudes, accepting a diminished role in society, even when their lived experiences contradict such narratives. Statements like "*It's time for me to step aside now*" or "*I can no longer do things as I used to*" reflect a resignation that reinforces the belief in the inevitability of personal decline. Such self-perceptions not only affect the individual but also shape broader societal attitudes, perpetuating the notion that aging equates to an irreversible loss of personhood.

Ageist attitudes—whether experienced or enacted—lead to poorer quality of life, reduced access to preventive healthcare, and inadequate medical treatment. Older individuals may be subjected to dismissive medical practices, including the denial of treatment or exclusion from clinical interventions deemed unnecessary due to their age. Furthermore, ageist misconceptions often overshadow positive attributes of individuals with dementia, reinforcing discriminatory practices, sometimes even without full awareness [22]. One striking example is therapeutic nihilism—the belief that there is little to no benefit in treating aging individuals, particularly those diagnosed with dementia. This perspective exacerbates systemic ageist stigma within healthcare and social services, severely limiting access to appropriate care. When aging is synonymous with frailty and chronic illness, healthcare professionals and caregivers may inadvertently adopt a pessimistic outlook that permeates geriatric facilities, particularly those serving individuals with dementia. Consequently, older adults with dementia continue to experience profound inequalities in receiving adequate support for daily activities compared to younger individuals with similar conditions.

Compounding this issue is the persistent violation of human rights that aged individuals—particularly those with dementia—often endure across various levels of interaction, from family dynamics to institutional policies. Following a dementia diagnosis, individuals are frequently excluded from decision-making processes, resulting in their specific needs being overlooked or dismissed. A particularly concerning consequence of this marginalization is the reduction of the person to their disease [23]. In such cases, the "demented" label supersedes their personal history, identity, and lived experiences. As a result, care systems focus primarily on managing the symptoms of dementia rather than addressing the holistic needs of the individual, leading to the misinterpretation of behaviors and the administration of inadequate interventions.

One of the gravest consequences of ageist stigma is its role in delaying dementia diagnosis. The widespread misconception that cognitive decline and loss of autonomy are inherent aspects of aging contributes to the significant underdiagnosis of dementia. Estimates suggest that approximately two-thirds of individuals with dementia receive a diagnosis only in the later stages of the disease, and as many as half remain undiagnosed entirely [24]. The lack of early detection poses a major challenge, particularly given that an early diagnosis offers substantial benefits—not only in terms of quality of life but also in economic and social dimensions, as well as in reducing caregiver burden.

Several factors contribute to delays in dementia diagnosis [25–27]. Among the primary reasons is a lack of awareness regarding the distinction between normal aging and pathological cognitive decline. Additionally, many individuals experiencing early symptoms categorically refuse to acknowledge their condition, avoid discussing concerns with family members, or hesitate to seek specialist consultations due to fear, stigma, or denial. The reluctance to pursue a diagnosis is often exacerbated by the prevailing societal belief that cognitive and behavioral changes do not constitute a legitimate medical issue. Moreover, doubts about the effectiveness of medical interventions and concerns about the social consequences of being diagnosed with dementia further discourage individuals from seeking professional evaluation.

While an early diagnosis of dementia does not prevent disease progression, it plays a fundamental role in improving an individual's quality of life. Early detection allows for the establishment of supportive environments that foster autonomy, self-determination, and dignity throughout the disease trajectory. For individuals with dementia, receiving a timely diagnosis means having the opportunity to understand and make sense of their condition, engage in advance care planning, and explore potential pharmacological and non-pharmacological interventions that may slow cognitive decline.

Addressing the complexities of dementia diagnosis requires a comprehensive approach that considers individual, interpersonal, and cultural factors. Only by recognizing these multifaceted challenges can we mitigate the risk of further alienating individuals with dementia and ensure that they receive the care and support necessary to maintain their dignity and well-being.

4. Toward a health-oriented approach to dementia

Luckily, there is growing evidence of a segment of the population that does not exhibit significant signs of resignation. Instead, they increasingly reaffirm self-determination, even after receiving a dementia diagnosis. The approach proposed here seeks to move beyond the meanings perpetuated by ageism and its derivatives, advocating for the fundamental "right to age." This right emphasizes the active participation of individuals in shaping personal and societal transformations through reciprocal relationships and shared commitments. The goal is to foster an inclusive environment where everyone, including individuals with dementia, can find the necessary conditions to realize their full potential.

A critical aspect of this perspective involves careful attention to the physical, cultural, and social contexts in which aging unfolds. Equally important is recognizing the opportunities available to each individual, shaped by their unique life history, in order to support the fullest expression of their personal identity. The aging process comprises a complex interplay between well-being, frailty, and pathology, which cannot be reduced to predetermined standards.

Thus, it is crucial to assess from the outset not only the cognitive reserve that a given individual possesses but also the environmental and social contexts in which they are embedded. This understanding is fundamental for designing psychological and educational interventions that promote well-being, facilitate life trajectories, and empower the surrounding community. Key elements of this transformative approach include, beyond the necessity of early diagnosis, the right to age in place, the opportunity for individual empowerment, and the presence of caregivers equipped with empathetic competencies to ensure meaningful cohabitation and support.

4.1 The exigency of "aging in place" and of a dementia-friendly community development

In recent years, the concept of aging in place has gained widespread recognition. It refers to the ability to remain in one's own home, despite an increasing need for support due to significant age-related changes that lead to greater frailty [28]. In this context, one strand of urban planning and design that promotes sustainable and participatory citizenship focuses on conceptualizing and developing urban infrastructure and services that are increasingly accessible and inclusive for individuals with dementia (see Dementia-Friendly Communities [29]).

Dementia-Friendly Communities are designed to ensure active participation in society by fostering the inclusion of individuals with dementia through tailored educational and training initiatives that engage all community members. These communities go beyond the mere provision of care services; instead, they adopt a holistic and proactive approach that sustains meaningful social engagement and empowerment for individuals with dementia. By doing so, they create a network of support that enables individuals to remain active contributors to their communities, despite cognitive decline.

This shift represents a significant advancement in dementia care, and many countries are now investing in the development of Dementia-Friendly Communities. However, these initiatives risk being insufficient if they remain predominantly confined to assistive care models and fail to incorporate a fundamental rethinking of dementia itself. Genuine community empowerment—and, consequently, the true inclusion of individuals with dementia—requires the implementation of educational programs targeted at citizens of all ages. This means not only engaging older adults but also integrating science-based dementia education into school curricula and public awareness campaigns.

A truly Dementia-Friendly approach must prioritize widespread knowledge dissemination to differentiate between dementia and non-pathological aging, thereby fostering a more informed and inclusive society.

4.2 The benefits of early and differential diagnosis

For decades, scientific research has emphasized the importance of distinguishing aging from disease, highlighting how the irreversible changes associated with advancing age are not necessarily disabling. Nevertheless, despite growing awareness, many individuals continue to conflate cognitive decline with aging, failing to differentiate between dementia—certain forms of which result in cognitive impairment—and the natural, non-pathological changes in cognitive functioning that occur in later life. This misconception, which aligns with the broader issue of ageism, reflects persistent societal stigma surrounding aging and cognitive health.

From a biological perspective, the transition from cognitive normality to full-blown dementia is not demarcated by a clear threshold (see, for example, the challenges in defining Mild Cognitive Impairment [MCI]). This underscores the need for scientifically grounded public education on the complex interplay between aging and dementia. Widespread dissemination of accurate information—through educational initiatives in public spaces—can foster a shared understanding, serving as the foundation for more inclusive and Dementia-Friendly Communities.

Only in recent decades, due to advances in clinical research and neurodiagnostic techniques, has it become possible to delineate how the aging nervous system undergoes structural and functional modifications, ultimately contributing to various forms of dementia. Today, the term dementia has taken on a clinically precise meaning, referring to a syndrome characterized by a progressive decline in cognitive functions severe enough to interfere with social and occupational activities. This deterioration may also affect personality, emotions, and behavior, leading to a gradual loss of autonomy [30]. Older adults diagnosed with a form of dementia typically exhibit significantly impaired cognitive and functional abilities, affecting not only their own lives but also those of their primary caregivers, whose routines and responsibilities undergo profound transformations.

Individuals experiencing significant alterations in cognitive function must be able to recognize whether these changes are part of normal aging or indicative of a neurodegenerative condition. Consequently, seeking specialized medical consultation becomes essential in determining whether cognitive changes are within expected age-related variability or are suggestive of an emerging dementia-related pathology. An early neuropsychological assessment plays a pivotal role in identifying the initial clinical manifestations of cognitive impairment and facilitating differential diagnosis, allowing for the distinction between various neurodegenerative disorders. Furthermore, clarifying the differences between aging-related cognitive changes and dementia syndromes is critical for implementing effective interventions aimed at slowing disease progression, alleviating symptoms, and ultimately enhancing the quality of life for both individuals with dementia and their caregivers.

For all these reasons, it is imperative that society supports individuals in seeking a diagnosis free from stigma, ensuring that early detection becomes a pathway to timely intervention and comprehensive care.

4.3 Quality of life and individual empowerment

Ensuring that individuals, even those diagnosed with dementia, experience a high-quality aging process requires the promotion of both knowledge and proactive actions that empower individuals to take control of their own health trajectories [31, 32]. This necessitates overcoming ageist stereotypes, which often assume that people with dementia are incapable of self-determination. However, just like any other individual, a person living with dementia should be encouraged—and supported in learning—on how to take responsibility for their own aging journey. They should also have the agency to make informed decisions that help them manage their condition more effectively [33]. In this regard, individuals must have the opportunity to develop a comprehensive understanding of dementia, including its characteristics and implications for their future [34]. Thus, they should be able to play an active role in selecting the most appropriate treatment options [35] and choosing among the care services available in their local community [36].

Beyond dementia, research on successful aging suggests that individuals who maintain a high quality of life are those who actively empower themselves by adopting self-respecting lifestyles. This approach is referred to as empowering aging, which emphasizes that individuals, regardless of their health status, should be encouraged to seek personal growth, meaningful experiences, and fulfilling relationships, thereby exercising self-determination over their aging process. Similarly, when prioritizing quality of life despite dementia, the concept of empowerment requires a shift from a task-oriented care model, which focuses primarily on disease management, toward person-centered care, which places the individual at the core of all interventions. Such an approach enables individuals to maintain greater control over their health-related decisions and actions [37].

Of course, it is essential to recognize that empowerment in dementia differs from that of individuals experiencing typical aging. Cognitive, emotional, and behavioral changes associated with dementia inevitably affect decision-making abilities and motivations for self-determination. However, this does not diminish the fundamental importance of empowerment in supporting individuals with dementia to continue playing an active role in their own lives. Unfortunately, the role of first-person involvement in healthcare decisions is often overlooked in dementia care. Yet, research highlights that enabling individuals with dementia to participate in decision-making regarding their treatment and care pathways not only helps them preserve their sense of autonomy and competence but also serves as a motivational factor in maintaining engagement with life [38, 39]. Even when the risk of suboptimal decision-making is high and external support is required, fostering opportunities for empowerment can still lead to meaningful shared experiences between individuals with dementia and their caregivers [40].

In this context, understanding a person's life history, beliefs, values, preferences, and needs becomes crucial in shaping an empowerment-oriented approach. Such an approach aligns with the principles of Dementia-Friendly Communities, which emphasize inclusivity and social engagement. Creating opportunities for participation helps combat the social isolation and stigma often associated with dementia. Moreover, promoting equal partnerships in decision-making [41] encourages individuals with dementia to remain socially active and maintain a shared identity with others who also value empowerment, despite their condition [42]. The ability to make autonomous life choices, even when relying on external support, remains a cornerstone of empowerment in dementia care. This approach ensures that individuals can maximize their life potential while maintaining a sense of dignity and control.

Recent studies have demonstrated that empowerment in dementia leads to positive changes in quality of life and well-being, fostering greater self-confidence, self-esteem, and dignity throughout the progression of the disease [43, 44]. The ability to feel respected, valued, and included in decisions regarding one's care reinforces a sense of self [45, 46] and helps individuals maintain their social identity, despite cognitive decline [38].

While there may be debate about whether improved quality of life is a direct outcome of empowerment, or whether quality of life itself contributes to greater autonomy and self-determination, empowerment in aging must remain a central objective in dementia care. Ultimately, empowerment is a dynamic process, shaped by the interaction between the individual and their environment. Thus, the broader social context must acknowledge its role in facilitating true empowerment. This can only be achieved through a comprehensive understanding of the real needs of individuals with dementia and the development of services and policies that promote self-determination, rather than simply offering passive assistance. The principles of Dementia-Friendly Communities serve as a powerful framework for fostering empowerment, reducing stigma, and transforming societal perceptions of dementia.

4.4 Well-being and empathetic caregiving

The caregiving relationship—whether established through professional figures (e.g., healthcare professionals), family caregivers, or the broader social context (e.g., the community)—plays a crucial role in influencing the empowerment process of individuals living with dementia. In this context, reference is often made to widely recognized approaches such as the Gentlecare model [47] and the Validation method [48], which provide caregivers with strategies to allocate adequate time for relational engagement, offer continuous positive feedback to the needs of individuals with dementia, and, ultimately, establish an empathetic connection [49].

More specifically, the ability to adopt another person's perspective and achieve emotional attunement with the care recipient are key components of empowerment.

Perspective-taking is broadly defined as the cognitive process through which caregivers gain insight into how individuals with dementia might perceive and experience the world. This form of perspective-taking is often an imaginative exercise, wherein caregivers symbolically or metaphorically "step into the shoes" of the person with dementia to develop a multidimensional understanding of their thoughts and emotions. This competency, known as *social perspective-taking* (or *role-playing*), is typically acquired during late adolescence and has been associated with altruistic behaviors, increased likelihood of providing assistance, and reduced stress levels in observers witnessing another person's suffering.

If the primary objective of a caregiver is to ensure a high quality of life for the person being cared for, their efforts can only be deemed effective if they can accurately assess whether the individual has truly achieved a satisfactory level of well-being. Since caregivers do not personally experience the cognitive changes associated with dementia, they must actively engage in an "other-than-self" perspective when evaluating the well-being of those they assist. However, this task is inherently challenging, as it is difficult for caregivers to fully grasp what is essential for individuals with dementia to experience a sense of fulfillment.

Notably, research indicates that family caregivers often underestimate the quality of life of their relatives with dementia compared to self-assessments provided by the individuals themselves. Moreover, informal caregivers who are significantly younger than their care recipients tend to exhibit greater discrepancies in their evaluations of well-being compared to older caregivers. In contrast, older informal caregivers tend to provide more favorable assessments of the quality of life of the person with dementia [50]. One possible explanation for this variation is the differing perspectives on well-being held by individuals at different stages of life. It is important to note, however, that when caregivers are asked to evaluate the quality of life of individuals with dementia based on objective experiences and observable health-related symptoms—rather than on subjective thoughts or perceptions—their assessments tend to align more closely with those of the individuals receiving care. This finding supports the notion that perceptions of quality of life are inherently subjective.

Perspective-taking is particularly critical in dementia caregiving because, while cognitive decline may reduce situational awareness for the person with dementia, the caregiver's goal remains to provide the highest possible quality of life. However, when there is a discrepancy between the perspectives of the caregiver and the care recipient, this misalignment may lead to persistent frustration for the caregiver or a lack of recognition by the person with dementia that their support needs are being met. If caregiving efforts focus primarily (or exclusively) on actions that do not align with the individual's subjective sense of well-being, the person receiving care may not experience meaningful improvements in their quality of life.

Thus, for a caregiving relationship in the context of dementia to be truly characterized as "high-quality," an optimal level of empathy must be achieved. Only through this empathetic attunement can the quality of care be enhanced while simultaneously promoting the well-being of both caregivers and care recipients [51].

5. From theory to action: Some ongoing projects to improve caring for people with dementia

The purpose of this section is to present as an example some of the most significant projects that, through applied research, seek to translate the theoretical framework outlined thus far into practical implementation. Most of these initiatives are ongoing and involve scholars and early career researchers affiliated with the CHL—Centre for Healthy Longevity at the University of Bergamo. The majority of the presented projects interpolate more than one of the dimensions described above, but they are described here grouped according to the dimension considered to be their primary focus.

5.1 Fostering communities to be dementia friendly

As previously discussed, enhancing the quality of life for individuals living with dementia requires the presence of an urban community that is well educated in the principles of inclusion. Such a community should actively foster a "friendly" environment around individuals with dementia, ensuring not only that they are not isolated but also that they are fully accepted and able to continue expressing their individuality, despite their condition. The foundational vision behind the development of these communities' centers on the person with dementia as an individual recognized for their competencies and capabilities rather than being solely defined by their pathology.

A Dementia-Friendly Community (DFC) [52] is an urban environment in which every member, in both personal and professional capacities, learns to recognize what is expected of them and how they can contribute to supporting individuals who, while experiencing cognitive decline, should not be excluded from community life. A DFC is not exclusively composed of healthcare professionals and family members of individuals with cognitive frailty; rather, it is a community where all members play a role in facilitating meaningful life experiences for people with dementia—whether they are clients, neighbors, or acquaintances. In such a community, sales personnel are trained to assist individuals who may struggle with decision-making while shopping, financial and legal advisors take into account the challenges their clients may face in evaluating risks, and public transportation operators develop an increased awareness of and patience for those who may become spatially or temporally disoriented. More broadly, every community member who interacts with a person with dementia does not merely perceive them as a "forgetful, non-autonomous individual" but rather as a person to be understood and embraced in their entirety.

Thus, a DFC is an urban community that is informed about dementia, unafraid of it, and fully aware of how to actively contribute to enabling people with dementia to continue leading fulfilling lives. This approach requires a fundamental shift—from a welfare-based model to one that places the individual at the center, recognizing and valuing their agency. However, this transition is contingent upon one essential factor: the ability of the environment, the community, and the broader social context to undergo a profound cultural shift.

To facilitate this cultural transformation, the Dementia Friendly Italia project was launched in 2016 at the University of Bergamo and has since continued as a Public Engagement initiative within the CHL—Centre for Healthy Longevity. The project seeks to educate urban communities and foster a shared commitment between citizens and individuals with dementia in creating inclusive environments that respect and accommodate diverse needs. One of its primary objectives is to raise public awareness about dementia, dispelling the misconception that it is an inevitable component of aging or that it is exclusively linked to Alzheimer's disease. Furthermore, the project aims to provide the general public with deeper insight into the lived experiences of individuals with dementia.

To this end, educational initiatives have been organized in schools, municipalities, religious institutions, and professional associations (e.g., retailers, restaurant and bar operators, office employees, etc.). These activities equip various sectors of society with the necessary knowledge and tools to initiate a cultural transition, reframing cognitive frailty and dementia as conditions that require adaptation and support rather than exclusion.

In the projects implemented across Bergamo and surrounding areas, particular emphasis has been placed on creating meaning through participation, which is considered the cornerstone of building a community that is not only efficient but, above all, effective in fostering genuine inclusivity. Instead of merely developing "dementia-friendly" facilities, the initiative has aimed to cultivate what philosopher Margaret Gilbert [53] describes as a collective subject—a community that acts not as a collection of individuals but rather as a unified entity.

Thus, the educational sessions have sought to create a shared commitment, fostering a "collective we" rather than enforcing top-down directives. The goal is not to impose change through institutional training but rather to facilitate and encourage a grassroots transformation, enabling communities to develop authentic and sustainable ways of integrating people with dementia into everyday life.

The small Dementia-Friendly Communities that have emerged within schools (from preschool to secondary education) and various urban areas have gradually become recognized social spaces, where the implications and responsibilities of inclusivity are both acknowledged and acted upon. These communities are now perceived as part of a shared social mission, redefining the way dementia is understood within the collective mindset.

Moreover, each of these communities has faced the challenge of mobilizing and sustaining participation among all members—including people with dementia—who are empowered to exercise agency in decision-making processes. The project has thus facilitated the development of genuinely inclusive Dementia-Friendly Communities, capable of ensuring autonomy in life trajectories and safeguarding the rights of individuals living with dementia. In doing so, these communities contribute to breaking down social stigma while simultaneously reinforcing a sense of personal self-efficacy among individuals with dementia.

5.2 Identifying frailty to facilitate early dementia diagnosis: Bergamo and the "aged of the future"

To assess the aging potential of Bergamo's population—currently within the old-adult (55–65 years) or early old (65–75 years) age segments—a survey has been initiated to detect early psycho-cognitive frailty in these groups. The primary objective is to direct individuals, where necessary, toward early diagnosis programs, as well as to initiate the pre-frail population to psycho-education projects. These interventions are informed by recent evidence [54] and aim to promote protective lifestyle modifications that may reduce future dementia risk. Collectively, these population-based strategies are designed to guide participants toward a trajectory of quality aging. Beyond addressing care needs, the study identifies the resources and potential of the soon-to-age population through standardized questionnaires (assessing cognitive, emotional, and relational dimensions) alongside semi-structured interviews exploring subjective perspectives on aging and coping strategies for the transition into old age.

The project's innovative approach lies in its lifespan-centered assessment of individual potential and limitations, moving beyond a narrow focus on old age. This broader perspective helps discern how these factors may constrain or facilitate successful aging while enabling early dementia detection. By monitoring developmental trajectories in adulthood, the intervention supports activities that foster successful aging. Recognizing the complexity of lifespan development—where certain trajectories may predispose individuals to future frailty—the project implements psycho-promotional measures to encourage health-supportive behaviors before clinical manifestations emerge.

The intervention's objectives and methodologies are grounded not only in general aging dimensions derived from literature but are also tailored to critical or high-potential areas identified through local cultural and needs analyses. The methodology combines community-based work, alternating between individual and group interventions. Techniques include psychological empowerment, cognitive training, physical activity, socialization initiatives, and reinforcement of socio-health networks, all selected based on questionnaire and interview analyses.

The project delineates four prospective aging trajectories for enrolled participants [55]: (1) Future seniors who can maintain optimal psychophysical functioning, full autonomy, and maximized quality of life; (2) Future seniors who can grow old with psychophysical health, minor compensable limitations, and good quality of life; (3) Future seniors at risk of psychophysical frailty, experiencing substantial limitations in daily autonomy and quality of life; (4) Future seniors susceptible to age-related psychophysical illnesses (e.g., chronic or neurodegenerative diseases, depression), significantly impairing autonomy and quality of life.

Ongoing psycho-educational interventions are customized to each group's needs. The 12-month psycho-promotional program employs hybrid (online/in-person) individual and group sessions, informational materials (including multimedia), and experiential methods (e.g., role-playing, immersive virtual reality), following Bartholomew's implementation model [56]. Interventions aim to preserve optimal aging through healthy longevity strategies; enhance aging trajectories by improving autonomy; equip frail individuals with protective and compensatory strategies; and support them in pursuing early clinical/diagnostic measures to improve quality of life, despite dementia.

By envisioning Bergamo's aging future, this project seeks to identify individual-environment dynamics that either foster successful aging or optimize early dementia diagnosis through psycho-education—enabling residual function preservation before frailty becomes disabling. It advances healthy aging by framing old age as a continuum shaped by earlier life stages. The dual-purpose interventions aim to enhance well-being while educating participants on necessary adjustments for healthier aging. In addition, the project intends to empower people in adulthood to become the main actors in the design of quality aging (even in dementia), counteracting the stereotypical idea that aging is only and exclusively an age of loss, on which improvement interventions cannot be implemented.

5.3 Empowerment by the sea: The sailing experience of people living with dementia on Nave Italia

Aligned with the principle of centering individuals with dementia and empowering them in their lived experiences with the disease, the project "Psychological

Well-being for Elderly People with Dementia through Cruise Therapy" was conducted aboard Nave Italia, the world's largest brigantine. This initiative brought together people with dementia, educators and psychologists from the University of Bergamo, and the Italian Navy crew, facilitated by the foundation Tender to Nave Italia (TTNI, https://www.naveitalia.org/). For years, TTNI has combated prejudice against disability and social marginalization by promoting empowerment projects for vulnerable populations. Annually, it enables diverse groups to embark on weeklong voyages along the Mediterranean, living collectively as crew members—sharing cabins, performing navigation tasks, maintaining the deck, and managing meals—thus reinforcing agency in daily life, even within an exceptional context. This approach underscores the need to empower people in their everyday life (albeit in an exceptional context) in every trajectory of their growing old, including that of growing old with dementia.

During our onboarding as crew of University scholars and aged individuals, 24 people (70–90 years old) with moderate cognitive impairment resulting from neurodegenerative pathology were involved. The main objective of the cruise was to integrate the experience of sailing with moments of non-pharmacological interventions aimed at enhancing emotional well-being, social engagement, and psychomotor abilities. Additionally, a mixed-methods (quantitative-qualitative) design assessed whether the cruise experience improved psycho-emotional well-being and quality of life (QoL), informing future interventions that combine sailing with empowerment through travel [57].

To this end, the weeklong journey on Nave Italia necessitated a planning that covered the entire calendar year. In the pre-shipment phase (January–August), the methodology and all research materials were predisposed, as well as the quantitative-qualitative statistical designs for evaluating the effectiveness of the proposed treatments were defined. A training was also provided to educators for the administration of non-pharmacological interventions and Nave Italia method during the boarding phase. Not least, a recruitment and support action were carried out to accompany elderly persons with dementia and caregivers to the ship travel experience. In the post-boarding phase (September–December), data on psychophysical, emotional, autonomy, and quality-of-life status, collected before and during the boarding phase, were processed and evaluated in relation to the psycho-emotional well-being and quality-of-life status assessed immediately after the cruise experience and with a 3-month follow-up. These data were also compared with the same evaluations carried out with a control group of similar age and socioeconomic status that did not board the brigantine.

About the results achieved by comparing the pre- and post-boarding questionnaires given to our "sailors" versus a control group, we observed a slight improvement in cognitive level (assessed by the Mini Mental State Examination scale), an improvement in symptoms of depression (assessed by the Geriatric Depression Scale), and a substantial improvement in perceived quality of life (assessed by the World Health Organization WHOQOL scale). However, the small, heterogeneous sample (varying in age, gender, education, and diagnosis) necessitates cautious interpretation. Despite this, observed emotional gains, partially restored autonomy, and heightened self-determination suggest that the project holds promise as an empowerment strategy for people with dementia. Future iterations with larger experimental and control groups are planned to further validate these outcomes.

5.4 Virtual reality based first-person perspective on living with dementia

To foster a deeper understanding of the lived experiences of individuals with dementia and promote empathic attunement among caregivers, an innovative educational-experiential intervention was developed using immersive virtual reality (VR) technology. The ViveDe project (www.vivede.it) employs 360° videos, accessible via VR headsets, to simulate first-person perspectives of common daily challenges faced by people with dementia—such as shopping, cooking, dining out, or visiting a doctor. These videos, available on YouTube with full 360° explorability (x/y axis), allow users, including those unfamiliar with dementia, to virtually embody the cognitive and sensory disruptions associated with the condition.

Beyond enhancing caregiver comprehension of their care recipients' behaviors, the project aims to engage a broader audience—including those typically disinterested in dementia-related issues—in critical reflection on the motivations behind behaviors often perceived as challenging (e.g., wandering, hoarding, or food refusal). To evaluate the efficacy of this immersive experience in cultivating empathy, participants were interviewed before and after the VR session regarding their perceptions of dementia-related needs and their willingness to adopt a collaborative caregiving role. Data indicate that ViveDe significantly influences how both caregivers and non-professionals perceive dementia and its symptomatic manifestations [58].

In this way, the project seems to succeed in minimizing the idea that assistance should be delegated to welfare professionals (such as hospitals or nursing homes). At the same time, it also seems to succeed not only to make family members understand how to better accommodate their caregiver's demands, but also to people not directly involved (e.g., neighbors, shopkeepers, etc.) on how to include people with dementia more effectively within a Dementia Friendly Community. People who benefit from the ViveDe experience, in fact, become more aware of how an everyday activity (like buying bread and fruit in a neighborhood shop) can be a simple or very complicated challenge for a person with dementia strictly depending on the empathetic or not empathetic attitude of the others around them (e.g., the shop manager or the other customers). It is this shift that enables people with dementia to feel empowered to live a part of their lives independently, thereby counteracting part of their cognitive and motor decline.

The novelty of ViveDe lies in its integration of transformative VR technology with a psychological framework prioritizing quality of life in dementia care. It expands conventional educational paradigms by redefining autonomy and emphasizing the collective effort required for inclusive urban support systems. Crucially, the project underscores that the needs of individuals with dementia extend beyond basic physiological and safety requirements to encompass higher-order needs—social belonging, esteem, and self-actualization. By facilitating first-person experiential learning, ViveDe advocates for a paradigm shift from a narrow "care-as-custodial" model to one that actively upholds the self-determination and dignity of individuals with dementia.

Building on these findings, ViveDe is being adapted into a psycho-educational program for family caregivers of newly diagnosed individuals [59]. Through weekly VR-assisted training and discussion sessions, caregivers develop cognitive empathy by virtually assuming the perspective of the person with dementia. This approach aims to enhance caregivers' role awareness while concurrently improving the quality of life for both caregivers and care recipients.

Author details

Francesca Morganti
Department of Human and Social Sciences, CHL—Centre for Healthy Longevity, University of Bergamo, Bergamo, Italy

*Address all correspondence to: francesca.morganti@unibg.it

References

[1] Borges MK et al. Frailty as a predictor of cognitive disorders: A systematic review and meta-analysis. Frontiers in Medicine. 2019;**6**:26. DOI: 10.3389/fmed.2019.00026

[2] Godin J et al. Dynamics of frailty and cognition after age 50 why it matters that cognitive decline is mostly seen in old age. Journal of Alzheimer's Disease. 2017;**58**:231-242

[3] Wallace L et al. Investigation of frailty as a moderator of the relationship between neuropathology and dementia in Alzheimer's disease: A cross-sectional analysis of data from the rush memory and aging project. The Lancet Neurology. 2019;**18**:177-184

[4] Satz P. Brain reserve capacity on symptom onset after brain injury: A formulation and review of evidence for threshold theory. Neuropsychology. 1993;**7**:273-295

[5] Morganti F, Negri I. How cognitive reserve could protect from dementia? An analysis of everyday activities and social behaviors during lifespan. Brain Sciences. 2025;**5**. DOI: 10.3390/brainsci15060652

[6] Nyberg L et al. Memory aging and brain maintenance. Trends in Cognitive Sciences. 2012;**16**:292-305

[7] Fjell AM et al. Brain changes in older adults at very low risk for Alzheimer's disease. Journal of Neuroscience. 2013;**33**:8237-8242

[8] Park DC, Reuter-Lorenz P. The adaptive brain: Aging and neurocognitive scaffolding. Annual Review of Psychology. 2009;**60**:173-196

[9] Nyberg L, Pudas S. Successful memory aging. Annual Review of Psychology. 2019;**70**:219-243

[10] Sachdev PS et al. Classifying neurocognitive disorders: The DSM-5 approach. Nature Reviews Neurology. 2014;**10**:634-642

[11] American Psychiatric Association. DSM-5. Manuale Diagnostico e Statistico dei Disturbi Mentali. Milano: Raffaello Cortina; 2013

[12] Cacciaglia R et al. Effects of apoe-ε4 allele load on brain morphology in a cohort of middle-aged healthy individuals with enriched genetic risk for Alzheimer's disease. Alzheimer's & Dementia. 2018;**14**:902-912

[13] Stern Y. Cognitive reserve. Neuropsychologia. 2009;**47**:2015-2028

[14] Stern Y et al. A task-invariant cognitive reserve network. NeuroImage. 2018;**178**:36-45

[15] Franke K et al. Estimating the age of healthy subjects from T1-weighted MRI scans using kernel methods: Exploring the influence of various parameters. NeuroImage. 2010;**50**:883-892

[16] Nyberg L, Wåhlin A. The many facets of brain aging. eLife. 2020;**9**. DOI: 10.7554/eLife.56640

[17] World Health Organization. World Report on Ageing and Health. 2015. Available from: https://apps.who.int/iris/handle/10665/186463

[18] Woo J. Frailty, successful aging, resilience, and intrinsic capacity: A cross-disciplinary discourse of the aging process. Current Geriatrics Reports. 2019;**8**:67-71

[19] Butler RN. Ageism: Another form of bigotry. The Gerontologist. 1969;**9**:243-246

[20] Lamont RA, Swift HJ, Abrams D. A review and meta-analysis of age-based stereotype threat: Negative stereotypes, not facts, do the damage. Psychology and Aging. 2015;**30**:180-193

[21] Levy BR et al. Ageism amplifies cost and prevalence of health conditions. The Gerontologist. 2018;**60**(1):174-181

[22] Nelson TD. Ageism: Prejudice against our feared future self. Journal of Social Issues. 2005;**61**:207-221

[23] Kitwood T. Dementia Reconsidered: The Person Comes First. London: Open University Press; 1997

[24] Gauthier S et al. World Alzheimer Report 2021: Journey through the Diagnosis of Dementia. London: Alzheimer's Disease International; 2021

[25] Perry-Young L et al. How people come to recognise a problem and seek medical help for a person showing early signs of dementia: A systematic review and meta-ethnography. Dementia. 2018;**17**:34-60

[26] Mendez MF. Early-onset alzheimer disease and its variants. Continuum (Minneapolis, Minn). 2019;**25**:34-51

[27] Wei H, Masurkar A, Razavian N. On gaps of clinical diagnosis of dementia subtypes: A study of Alzheimer's disease and Lewy body disease. Frontiers in Aging Neuroscience. 2021;**15**:1149036. DOI: 10.1101/2021.05.05.21256720

[28] Greenfield EA. Using ecological frameworks to advance a field of research, practice, and policy on aging-in-place initiatives. The Gerontologist. 2012;**52**:1-12

[29] Hung L et al. Creating dementia-friendly communities for social inclusion: A scoping review. Gerontology and Geriatric Medicine. 2021;7:23337214211013596

[30] McKhann GM et al. The diagnosis of dementia due to Alzheimer's disease: Recommendations from the National Institute on Aging-Alzheimer's Association workgroups on diagnostic guidelines for Alzheimer's disease. Alzheimer's & Dementia. 2011;7:263-269. DOI: 10.1016/j.jalz.2011.03.005

[31] Morganti F. Psicologia Dell'invecchiamento e Qualità della vita. Salute, Fragilità e Demenza. Roma: Carocci Editore; 2022

[32] Morganti F. Longevity as a responsibility: Constructing healthy aging by enacting within contexts over the entire lifespan. Geriatrics. 2024;**9**(4):93. DOI: 10.3390/geriatrics9040093

[33] Read ST, Toye C, Wynaden D. Experiences and expectations of living with dementia: A qualitative study. Collegian. 2017;**24**:427-432

[34] Shelton EG, Orsulic-Jeras S, Whitlatch CJ, Szabo SM. Does it matter if we disagree? The impact of incongruent care preferences on persons with dementia and their care partners. The Gerontologist. 2018;**58**:556-566. DOI: 10.1093/geront/gnw202

[35] Watt JA, Goodarzi Z, Veroniki AA, Nincic V, Khan PA, Ghassemi M, et al. Comparative efficacy of interventions for aggressive and agitated behaviors in dementia: A systematic review and network meta-analysis. Annals of Internal Medicine. 2019;**171**:633-642. DOI: 10.7326/M19-0993

[36] Di Fiandra T, Canevelli M, Di Pucchio A, Vanacore N, Italian Dementia National Plan Working Group. The Italian dementia national

plan. Commentary. Annali dell'Istituto Superiore di Sanità. 2015;**51**:261-264. DOI: 10.4415/ANN_15_04_02

[37] World Health Organization. Programme on Mental Health: WHOQOL User Manual, 2012 Revision. 1998. Available from: https://apps.who.int/iris/handle/10665/77932

[38] McConnell T, Best P, Sturm T, Stevenson M, Donnelly M, Taylor BJ, et al. A translational case study of empowerment into practice: A realist evaluation of a member-led dementia empowerment service. Dementia. 2020;**19**:1974-1996

[39] Maki Y, Takao M, Hattori H, Suzuki T. Promoting dementia-friendly communities to improve the well-being of individuals with and without dementia. Geriatrics and Gerontology International. 2020;**20**:511-519. DOI: 10.1111/ggi.13896

[40] Alsawy S, Tai S, McEvoy P, Mansell W. 'It's nice to think somebody's listening to me instead of saying "oh shut up"'. People with dementia reflect on what makes communication good and meaningful. Journal of Psychiatric and Mental Health Nursing. 2019;**27**:151-161

[41] Hicks B, Innes A, Nyman S. Exploring the 'active mechanisms' for engaging rural-dwelling older men with dementia in a community technological initiative. Ageing and Society. 2020;**40**:1906-1938. DOI: 10.1017/S0144686X19000357

[42] Mmako NJ, Courtney-Pratt H, Marsh P. Green spaces, dementia and a meaningful life in the community: A mixed studies review. Health & Place. 2020;**63**:102344. DOI: 10.1016/j.healthplace.2020.102344

[43] Hebert CA, Scales K. Dementia friendly initiatives: A state of the science review. Dementia. 2017;**18**:1858-1895

[44] Whelan S, Teahan Á, Casey D. Fostering the resilience of people with dementia: A narrative literature review. Frontiers in Medicine. 2020;**25**(7):45. DOI: 10.3389/fmed.2020.00045

[45] Swall A, Ebbeskog B, Lundh Hagelin C, Fagerberg I. Stepping out of the shadows of Alzheimer's disease: A phenomenological hermeneutic study of older people with Alzheimer's disease caring for a therapy dog. International Journal of Qualitative Studies on Health and Well-Being. 2017;**12**:1. DOI: 10.1080/17482631.2017.1347013

[46] Phillipson L et al. Involvement of people with dementia in raising awareness and changing attitudes in a dementia friendly community pilot project. Dementia. 2018;**18**:2679-2694

[47] Jones M. Gentlecare: Changing the Experience of Alzheimer's Disease in a Positive Way. New Westminster, BC: Moyra Jones Resources, Hartley & Marks Publishers; 1999

[48] Feil N. Validation therapy. Geriatric Nursing. 1992;**13**:129-133

[49] Smith R, Ooms A, Greenwood N. Supporting people with young onset dementia and their families: An evaluation of a training course for care workers. Nurse Education in Practice. 2017;**27**:7-12. DOI: 10.1016/j.nepr.2017.08.007

[50] Arons AM et al. Quality of life in dementia: A study on proxy bias. BMC Medical Research Methodology. 2013;**13**:110. DOI: 10.1186/1471-2288-13-110

[51] Wijma AJ et al. Patient-centeredness in physiotherapy: What does it entail? A systematic review of qualitative studies. Physiotherapy Theory and Practice. 2017;**33**:825-840

[52] Morganti F. Le comunità Dementia Friendly. Verso L'inclusione delle Persone con Fragilità Cognitiva. Milano: FrancoAngeli; 2018

[53] Gilbert M. On Social Facts. Princeton: Princeton University Press; 1989

[54] Livingston G et al. Dementia prevention, intervention, and care: 2020 report of the lancet commission. The Lancet. 2020;**396**:413-446

[55] Gattuso M, Butti S, Benincá I, Greco A, Di Trani M, Morganti F. A structural equation model for understanding the relationship between cognitive reserve, autonomy, depression and quality of life in aging. International Journal of Environmental Research and Public Health. 2024;**21**:9. DOI: 10.3390/ijerph21091117

[56] Bartholomew LK, Parcel GS, Kok G, Gottlieb N. Planning Health Promotion Programs: An Intervention Mapping Approach. 2nd ed. San Francisco: Jossey-Bass; 2006

[57] Morganti F, Brignoli P, Gagliani M, Cornaglia FP. Rivedere la rotta nella demenza: Nave Italia per le persone anziane con fragilità cognitive. In: Atti del 23° Congresso Nazionale AIP-Associazione Italiana Psicogeriatria; Firenze; 13-15 Aprile 2023. Firenze: Congresso Nazionale AIPAssociazione Italiana Psicogeriatria; 2023

[58] Morganti F et al. Take the first-person perspective to become dementia friendly: The use of 360° video for experiencing everyday-life challenges with cognitive decline. Frontiers in Psychology. 2020;**11**:117. DOI: 10.3389/fpsyg.2020.01117

[59] Morganti F, Gattuso M, Singh Solorzano C, Bonomini C, Rosini S, Ferrari C, et al. Virtual reality-based psychoeducation for dementia caregivers: The link between caregivers' characteristics and their sense of presence. Brain Sciences. 2024;**14**:852